SICK
of
DOCTORS?

Then do something about it!

A PRESCRIPTION FOR PATIENT EMPOWERMENT

LORENE M. BURKHART

FOREWORD BY

WILLIAM NORCROSS, MD

THE CURTIS
PUBLISHING
COMPANY

ISBN-13: 978-0-9841806-0-8
ISBN-10: 0-9841806-0-5

Library of Congress Control Number: 2010922026

CONTENTS

FOREWORD

Sick of Doctors? A Prescription for Patient Empowerment by Lorene Burkhart is a powerful and important book that should be read by all Americans. It is powerful in the breadth of what is covered and the currency of the references used to inform the reader. It is important in that we are all patients and have a vital interest in understanding the physicians who care for us: What motivates them; how they are selected; how the systems developed that control them and us in the U.S.; and perhaps most important, how we can partner with good physicians to shape a better health-care system today.

Beyond helping us understand the medical profession, however, *Sick of Doctors?* describes practical ways we can recognize good doctors and good health systems, take increasing responsibility for our own health care, communicate effectively with our physicians, and partner with doctors to improve the quality and safety of the care delivered to us and those we love.

Since I graduated from medical school over three decades ago, health care has transformed radically in the United States. Scientific and technological advances have dramatically improved the quality of life for those with access to care, but for those with access to minimal care or no care, the double-headed Hydra of soaring costs coupled with our archaic system of employer-based health insurance leaves many of our citizens to suffer and die from easily treatable diseases. Even many of us with health insurance feel a sense of disenfranchisement and dissatisfaction with the organization and effectiveness of our care. A system of health care has evolved that lavishly rewards high-tech procedures, invests a large percentage of the overall expenditure on the last few months of patients' lives, and provides few or no incentives for physicians or patients to practice preventive health care. While no other nation on the face of the earth can rival our economic power or scientific ingenuity, neither is there a country that has evolved a health-care system that even remotely mirrors our frankly bizarre structure and values.

Through Ms. Burkhart's careful journalistic effort, you will understand the social, psychological, economic, and cultural factors that created the American health-care system and gain important insights into the potential remedies that will be needed to solve the challenges before us.

Ms. Burkhart shows us how to achieve this. The Era of the Passive Patient has passed. The successful patient recognizes that a team approach is necessary for the effective delivery of care, and that the patient is an empowered member of that team. You will learn how to seek, recognize, and retain a "good doctor." You will learn how to be comfortable communicating with your doctor and other members of the team. While it is unrealistic to expect that every patient will have graduated from medical school or nursing school, the successful patient will be compelled to learn about the diseases and natural processes affecting his or her body and accurately report symptoms, responses to medications, and all information that the health team needs to provide optimal care.

This book is very well written. Ms. Burkhart, an accomplished author, writes with clarity, power, and authority. No sentence is superfluous; each paragraph is interesting and informative.

I have read this book, learned from it, and enjoyed it immensely. Although all citizens should read it, if I could select one sub-group to "assign" it to, it would be the medical students throughout our land. It seems to me that the information contained herein would be extremely helpful to them in understanding the roots of our profession, the powerful forces that act on us now, and what they must do to be the kind of doctors that they want to be.

William Norcross, MD
Director of Physician Assessment and Clinical Education
University of California, San Diego
November 2009

INTRODUCTION

HUBERT D. McCORMICK, my great uncle, received his medical degree in 1908. He practiced in an era when doctors worked out of small offices, made house calls, and received no payment from insurance (which didn't exist then anyway). The family affectionately called him "Uncle Doc," which in itself, I believe, speaks volumes. In the century since Uncle Doc began his practice, the medical industry has evolved to where a number of doctors work out of small offices, make house calls, and receive no payment from insurance.

Wait. Did I say that right? Yes — medicine actually has come full cycle. Nowadays, many physicians are leaving large medical consortia and starting small practices tailored more to address patients' personal needs. The BIG catch is that only the affluent can afford the hefty fees for the services these doctors offer. As a small-town rural doctor, Uncle Doc (and his contemporaries) often accepted as payment a couple of chickens or a basket of fresh-from-the-field produce. Today's small-practice medics, however, need more than just a few dollars to satisfy their fiscal hunger.

Why are these doctors striking out on their own? Frustration certainly plays a pivotal role, a frustration equal to that of the patients who navigate the difficult bureaucracy of the medical system. Despite these hurdles, the field of medicine abounds with dedicated young men and women who enter medical school with a deep commitment to help humanity.

So what does that have to do with us — the patients?

Face it: Most of us are patients from the beginning of life until the end. A doctor's signature appears on both birth and death certificates. What happens in the interim, however — our overall long-term health — is more important to us than anything else in our life. Without good health we falter at work and play, or simply fail to function optimally in a meaningful way in our families.

I have been seen by at least fifty doctors in my seventy-plus years, starting with Uncle Doc, who brought me into the world. He retired in 1946, when I was twelve years old, and his services were missed sorely. Gone was the reliance on a man who was not just loved, but revered in the community. No one doubted his devotion to his patients' well-being. Folks in rural areas like where I grew up were born and usually died in their homes. In between they depended on grit and home remedies for health issues. One went to a doctor only when very sick, or for an emergency, such as a broken bone. After my uncle closed up his practice, a new health-care life began. Doctor visits now involved a drive to town for prearranged appointments with a physician who was a stranger, one who had yet to earn our respect and trust.

Treatments changed just as dramatically. Scientific research produced a plethora of miracle drugs: sulfa, penicillin, insulin. Events like births and deaths moved from the home to the hospital. Of course, the cost of medical treatment rose accordingly, as did the appearance of bills, which were expected to be paid in cold, hard, and sometimes not-so-abundant cash — a pay-as-you-go system, if you will.

For me, this was just the beginning of a tsunami of changes in how medicine is practiced. Along the way, I was misdiagnosed, treated disrespectfully, and ignored. I endured the loss of medical records in the course of referrals to specialists I didn't need to see, underwent and suffered through unnecessary surgical procedures performed by a drug-addicted doctor — and lost my belief in doctors' ability to comprehend the need for day-to-day wellness care versus intervention. I am not alone: I have talked with many others who shared similar experiences, and doubtless, other stories must be legion.

Years ago, when I was a housewife — unemployed outside the home and uninsured — patients who paid cash for medical services paid more than those with insurance. And I don't mean just a co-pay — the actual bill was more. Now that I've reached my Medicare years I'm even more shocked by sky-high hospital and physician charges

Introduction

that are then discounted because of the health-care plan. For example, my twenty-hour stint at Cleveland Clinic for cardiac arrhythmia was tagged at nearly five thousand dollars! Who knows what the hospital actually received for my observation and treatment after bartering was settled. Later, I thought of what kind of luxury suite in a five-star hotel I could have had for that figurative five thousand dollars.

Granted, expensive charges are not determined exclusively by doctors. Like the rest of us, they are just trying to make a living. Nevertheless, they frequently order a battery of unnecessary tests — each one ratcheting the bill up higher — that are prescribed defensively to avoid potential lawsuits for "missing" something during the exam. Also, you have to wonder how often doctors order procedures just because they can, spurred by a desire to "get under the hood" and tinker until everything — meaning the patient — is "fixed" to their satisfaction.

Is it really caring, or is it ego? I marvel at how some physicians seem to labor under a bit of a "Doctor God" complex. Have you heard the old joke about the difference between God and a doctor? At least God knows He is not a doctor. Plenty of arrogant physicians pander to us, roll their eyes when we aren't looking (and sometimes even when we are), and then hustle off to their next fifteen-minute appointment.

At the same time, I have no doubt that for every bad Doctor God at least one outstandingly good Doctor God exists. In honesty, the majority of the many doctors I've seen over the years were caring, respectful, and honest. One orthopedic surgeon even admitted that he could not work miracles; all he could do was offer information, write a prescription, and perform any needed surgery. Bravo! I profoundly appreciated his honesty and straightforwardness.

I now better understand the conventional medical system and also see a variety of "alternative medicine" providers who work to help me live "health-fully." Some doctors I visit for acute care or to maintain a status quo for certain existing ailments, not to mention routine screenings for the various maladies that plague mankind.

I wonder, though: What along the way changed our attitudes

toward health care and doctors' attitudes toward patient care in our country? Today, people are disturbed, dismayed, and disgusted by what has happened to patient care. In fact, many are downright mutinous; they don't like where things are or where they seem to be going. To understand how patient care has arrived at its current state over the century, it's important to know how that evolution occurred. History, after all, tends to repeat itself. If we listen, it also offers valuable lessons — lessons that help us avoid mistakes of the past, effect change, and take charge of our health care.

In today's medical world, it is up to each of us to maintain health on a daily basis and not be dependent on an all-powerful Doctor God to do it for us. The old days are over.

Chapter 1
Forget the Old Days

RECALLING THE IMPORTANT medical moments in my life — my birth and childhood illnesses, the births of my children, the deaths of my parents and husband — I am struck by how clearly the circumstances surrounding those events reflect the changes we've witnessed in doctors and the delivery of medical services in America over the past one hundred years. From home-based businesses, to powerful and well-organized institutions, the industry that provides those services in America has undergone an amazing transformation.

In any so-called "big story" the broadest facts are best conveyed by zeroing in on the smallest details. In order to paint a vividly human portrait of American health care, we share the individual stories of physicians and physician families throughout this book, including some of my own.

When my brothers and I were born between 1925 and 1936, children were often born at home, especially in rural areas. In most cases, the doctors who oversaw those births shared long-term relationships with the families they served. Family doctors were often revered, but they worked hard to deliver the best care they could for their patients. Although many assumed doctors were wealthy, most were simply middle- or upper-middle-class professionals who attended the same churches, patronized the same businesses, and walked the same streets as did the people they served.

Our family doctor was truly a member of the family — my father's uncle Hubert D. McCormick, a starched and proper physician whom we all referred to as "Uncle Doc." For my birth, Uncle Doc made the seven-mile trip from his office in Vincennes, Indiana, to our family farm, just as he had and would for the births of each of my mother's four children. He prepared his instruments, delivered and cleaned the child, washed up in the large kitchen sink, returned to my mother's bedside to make sure she and her new baby were resting safely, then climbed back into his car and returned to town to see his other patients.

For routine matters of health, we made the trip to town. Uncle Doc's office was like any physician's workplace at that time. It occupied two rooms in the LaPlante Building in downtown Vincennes. Lettered on the opaque glass pane of the wooden door was my uncle's name. His daughter, Betty, when not in school, served as his receptionist; otherwise, he handled office duties himself. A small waiting room held a few straight chairs and a floor lamp or two — no glossy houseplants or magazines. To entertain yourself while waiting, you could look out the window at the traffic passing by on Second Street, stare at your shoes, and wonder what would happen to you after you crossed the hall into the inner sanctum of his office and sat opposite him under the glare of the light reflector he wore strapped around his forehead.

Uncle Doc's examining room was all business. Glass-paned cabinets lined the walls. A dark examining table with stiff leather upholstery draped in a crisp white sheet was the centerpiece of the room, and the atmosphere was set by the silvery glitter of medical instruments and the equally sharp smell of antiseptics and alcohol. Like the diploma he proudly displayed on the wall behind his large, uncluttered desk, the office itself announced my uncle's authority as a member of an elite group of professionals who maintained a uniquely intimate relationship with the clients they served. I was proud to be the niece of such an important and respected man.

Uncle Doc's downtown office also reflected a growing trend among doctors in even the most rural areas of the nation. When he graduated from the Indiana University School of Medicine (IUSM) in 1908, medicine was still largely a domestic practice in most parts of Indiana, centered on treating patients in their homes or in the physician's home-based office. As the century advanced, many doctors moved their practices into professional offices and general hospitals. House calls faded to a distant memory. At the same time, the American Medical Association (AMA) spearheaded a movement to professionalize the field of medicine by controlling the education and licensing of practicing physicians.

That effort was firmly rooted in economics. Throughout most of the nineteenth century, many doctors earned less than the average manufacturing laborer. By 1900, competition and quackery were rampant; various unorthodox health practices, such as homeopathy, osteopathy, and mind-control, attracted devoted followers. "Snake-oil" salesmen traveled freely about the country peddling "patent" medicines, and midwives and healers were common in many parts of the nation. The AMA's push for state licensure was unsuccessful in consolidating power among traditional medical practitioners. In the immediate wake of the rulings, numerous commercial medical schools popped up around the country — many little more than medical diploma mills. Even the best medical schools remained unregulated and could freely determine their own curriculum and admission standards.

My uncle began medical school without a high-school diploma. Even so, his training was much more extensive than many contemporaries. In 1901, when eighteen years old, Hubert McCormick enrolled in a two-year teaching course at Vincennes University. After teaching for a year, he entered IUSM. Upon graduation in 1908, he interned for one year at the school's dispensary and the Wabash Railroad Hospital in Peru, Indiana, before returning to Vincennes to take over the practice of a retiring physician.

GOOD-BYE HOUSE CALLS, HELLO HOSPITALS

By the time Uncle Doc saw his first patient, the AMA was making headway to reform medical education practices and to organize and promote doctors as an exclusive and well-regulated body of science-based professionals. Schools were now required to house specific types of laboratories and equipment for medical trainees or risk losing the ability to grant licenses. As a result, many medical schools partnered with universities and state colleges to benefit from the funds these institutions had at their disposal; others, unable to afford the upgrades to their facilities, shut down.

At the same time, the AMA was able to bring more physicians into its organization via a series of internal legislative acts. By the 1920s, state boards assumed greater control over the entrance qualifications, training, and licensing process. That control, coupled with the decline in the number of medical schools and medical school graduates, resulted in an increase in power and prestige for the medical profession.

Doctors slowly began to enjoy greater wealth and status. In his Pulitzer Prize-winning book, *The Social Transformation of American Medicine,* Paul Starr wrote that at the turn of the twentieth century, physicians made between $750 and $1500 a year; by 1934 — the heart of the Great Depression, when most workers' yearly salary averaged about $990 — doctors earned more than *four times* that amount, just over $4,000. Analysts who compiled the figures concluded that the AMA's strict control over access to the field of medicine was the reason for the Depression-era spike in earnings.

Unfortunately, poor rural areas found it harder to attract and keep doctors, who gravitated toward the better-paying cities and urban areas. The drain left some rural families with nowhere to turn but to the unorthodox practitioners the AMA worked so hard to eliminate. The wide availability of patent medicines and other unproven (and sometimes dangerous) home cures led many households to self-medicate in the absence of either the availability or affordability of a trained doctor. Medical expenses — especially those associated with hospitalization — rose dramatically.

The loss of rural health-care options and the expense of increasingly complex technology converged to create a near-health-care crisis in the country. Many people simply stopped going to the doctor, and those who did seek medical help often couldn't pay their bills. Hospital admissions plummeted, and many outlying hospitals folded. To combat the trend, some hospitals banded together to offer medical service plans to local businesses and groups. This act marked the beginning of a radical change: the introduction of health insurance plans that would come to be known as Blue Cross and Blue Shield.

While you might think doctors would have been in favor of the idea of pay-for-service insurance, that wasn't the case. From the first rumblings of the notion, the AMA deeply opposed any type of subsidized medical service program, fearing third-party control of pricing and practices. The organization also feared that Blue Cross service plans would eventually become compulsory insurance, under the control of the federal government. As the Depression deepened, both hospitals and individuals — especially those in the middle class — clamored for health-care expense assistance. Nevertheless, when Franklin Roosevelt crafted the New Deal legislation that resulted in Social Security, he intentionally left out any provisions for national health-care assistance, knowing that opposition from the AMA and the nation's social conservatives could kill the entire package. Starr writes that in 1943, as the long-running debate about national health-care insurance continued, Roosevelt commented to a Senate committee chairman, "We can't go up against the State Medical Societies; we just can't do it."

But nothing could stop the growth of Blue Cross' direct-service plans, which were funded and managed by individual hospitals or groups of hospitals across the nation. If doctors wanted to practice medicine, they had to participate in insurance. The AMA set its own standards for participation in such plans, drawing a firm line between payments to hospitals and individual patients, and payments to physicians. But Blue Cross plans didn't fulfill the growing demand for medical payment assistance for non-hospital-related doctor services. As a result, insurance companies emerged to craft and offer such coverage. The AMA was leery of commercial insurance companies' influence. At the same time, Blue Cross organizations feared losing business to the private insurers, so in the mid-1940s, with the AMA's grudging cooperation, many states created their own plans for covering doctor visits and services, in or out of the hospital.

These plans were managed by boards of physicians and came to be known as Blue Shield.

By that time, advancements in medicine offered doctors unprecedented options for diagnosing and treating patients. By the 1940s, even small-town doctors like my uncle utilized a wide range of diagnostic tools such as microscopes, X-ray equipment, and electrocardiographs available in their offices and local hospitals. Better transportation and increased availability of general hospitals and organized clinics in urban areas afforded more doctors the opportunity to focus on a single specialty. The convergence of changes transformed the way we thought of doctors and how we, as patients, interacted with them.

Good-bye, Uncle Doc. The domestic days of medicine were fading fast and the practice of medicine was firmly institutionalized. In the first half of the century, people didn't go to the doctor unless they were seriously ill. By the late 1940s, regular medical visits and "checkups" were routine for most families. Hospitalization became a common solution for the treatment of illness and injury. We learned to trust ourselves to the care of strangers, specialists, and institutions. For most of us, our "medical relationship" was with the health-care industry, rather than the comforting, highly respected individual who once served as our family doctor.

Chapter 2
Understand the System

In 1957, when my first child was born, I received obstetric care — a medical specialty that became quite popular during the population boom following World War II. My husband and I were both recent graduates of Purdue University; we had little money and no regular doctor. But my husband's job at J.C. Penney did provide him with Blue Cross/Blue Shield insurance coverage, so I could afford to follow a friend's recommendation to see her obstetrician. After a series of monthly, then weekly visits, my delivery date arrived and I was admitted to the hospital in Lafayette. The birth was blessedly uneventful. After spending the normal recuperative period of five to six days in the hospital, my son and I were released to return home. I don't remember if my husband and I paid *any* expenses for my hospital stay — I don't think we could have, given our financial situation. Thank heaven for Blue Cross/Blue Shield!

The Blues Pay — Doctors Specialize and Doctor Groups Are Born

After World War II, many companies offered employees benefits through a Blue Cross/Blue Shield plan. Traditionally, most doctors across the country used a sliding scale for patient charges; poor people paid less, rich people paid more. But the insurance plans offered everybody the same benefits at the same price, making it a good deal for the middle and upper classes, but not so great for lower-income families with little money to spend for health care. It also made Blue Cross/Blue Shield a non-factor in labor negotiations, which took on a big role in the post-war American workforce economy. As a result, large manufacturing companies that wanted to attract workers began turning to customized, private insurance plans that could be used as a bargaining chip in hiring.

This development also wasn't so great for low-income families for another reason: generous health-care plans tended to drive up the costs of health services. It turned out to be a major boon for doctors, though, and helped launch the medical services industry in this country. Medical insurance plans provided a reliable source of income that didn't depend upon the ups and downs of a local economy, or the ability (and willingness) of individuals to pay their medical bills. Payment for services became a third-party affair, with little exchange between the two central players. That, coupled with the growing mobility of the American workforce, meant that a physician might have a longer relationship with an insurance provider than he did with the patient who held the insurance.

Back in 1957, I certainly had no opportunity to establish any kind of a doctor–patient relationship with my obstetrician (whose name I've forgotten). Like many young couples in America at that time, my husband and I were on the move. My second child was born in Cincinnati, Ohio, in 1960. I found a new obstetrician, who, during an office visit early in my eighth month of pregnancy, told me to go home, pack my bag, and go to the hospital, because I was going to have the baby within twenty-four hours. I wasn't having labor pains — heck, I hadn't even ordered my birth announcements! But I didn't dream of questioning the doctor, and so with little understanding of why the baby would come so soon (and with no physical warning signs), to the hospital I went.

Although no baby materialized that day, the next morning I was rushed to the delivery room, where my son arrived quickly, without any warning contractions or labor pains. My doctor wasn't even at the hospital, but it was a good thing that I had heeded his advice. Due to complications with the birth process itself, neither my son nor I would have survived if the birth had occurred outside the hospital. I saw that doctor a few times for follow-up, but then lost contact with him. Thus, I became a medical "customer," obediently following doctor's orders and drawing upon the services of a vast and ever-growing industry, about whose costs or workings I knew little — and cared even less.

Doctors were on the move, too, during the 1950s and '60s. After the successful development of the Salk vaccine for polio in 1955, Americans were giddy with enthusiasm and hope for medical research. Government funding for research institutions skyrocketed, and doctors flocked to the new facilities. The United States government assisted in building community hospitals, and medical schools grew at a tremendous pace to meet the demand for more practitioners. As new doctors were drawn to the newest hospitals, research facilities, and medical schools of America's cities, the exodus eroded the already dwindling patient base of urban general practitioners. Many older GPs migrated to the suburbs, joining their patients in the flight from urban areas.

Specialization began taking a toll on the supply of family doctors, too. Like my obstetrician, many physicians entered specializations that offered larger salaries and more prestige. Insurance payments to specialists were healthy, too, especially when their services involved surgical procedures. All of these forces combined to fuel the engine of medical-expense inflation, and to put the good old family GP on the endangered species list. Doctors in private practice were in demand. As the number of patients they saw each day increased, less time was spent with each one. Americans saw multiple specialists and consulted with a range of physicians in group practices, rather than relying on a single medical provider. Patients began to resent the sometimes brusque treatment they received from their doctors, who often seemed to treat patients as a necessary annoyance, rather than the heart of their practices — and the source of their ever-expanding incomes.

UNCLE SAM AND PRIVATE INSURERS ENTER THE PAY PICTURE

In the 1960s, even as the nation's economy boomed right along with medical funding, advancements, and facilities, Americans living in run-down inner-city neighborhoods or poor rural areas had limited access to any medical care. In response to a growing concern over the lack of community health care, citizens once again grappled with the idea of a national program to address the issue. In 1965, President Lyndon Johnson signed into law a three-part health-care assistance program: Medicare, a compulsory government-subsidized program of hospital insurance provided as a part of Social Security; a partially subsidized voluntary insurance program for paying physician costs; and Medicaid, which supplied federal assistance to states, specifically allocated to paying for the medical expenses of the poor.

Once again, the AMA and its members balked at the government's dabbling in the delivery of medical services. Nevertheless, they quickly became comfortable with the "gold mine" called Medicare, which set the standard for payment for medical services based on charges, rather than on an agreed-upon fee list. And because the cooperation of hospitals and doctors was essential for the program to succeed, the Social Security Administration also conceded to pay hospitals for costs and for depreciation of their assets. Government expenditures on health care ballooned, along with the costs of most medical services; hospital stays got longer and the number of "routine" procedures grew.

Not surprisingly, by the mid-1960s, people began to cast a jaundiced eye at the medical profession in general. The heartfelt enthusiasm and support most Americans felt for medical research in the early 1950s was replaced with growing suspicion and resentment as reports surfaced that some teaching hospitals and research facilities were conducting dangerous tests on unknowing patients. In 1966, the National Institutes of Health (NIH) reacted to public outrage at these reports and required researchers to establish review boards to evaluate the potential benefits and risks of research. But even then, peer review was trusted to regulate an important process in what had become a big-money industry.

Medicare, of course, was one of the last century's defining influences on American health care. As the nation's largest social insurance program, Medicare spending represents a huge investment on the part of the federal government and its people. According to health-care analyst Marc A. Rodwin, Medicare spent $4.2 billion on inpatient hospital care in 1970. Within a mere fourteen years, that amount rose to $39.7 billion. In response to these rapidly rising costs, Medicare changed its payment system, to pay hospitals set fees for services, with the fees determined by the patients' diagnoses. This system encouraged hospitals to limit expenditures, since they could keep any "extra" money within the standard payment. At the same time, more doctors were becoming part-owners of hospitals and clinics throughout the 1980s and '90s. As a result, many doctors shared financial interests with the hospitals in which they practiced, leading to concerns about conflicts of interest within the profession.

HMO Who?

The rising cost of medical care also resulted in changes in private insurance systems. Many employers began funneling their group health benefits into Health Maintenance Organizations — the HMOs we are so sadly familiar with today. HMOs, first proposed in the early 1970s, offered dramatically reduced costs in exchange for stricter control over health-care providers and procedures. By targeting a narrow range of providers for a large number of enrollees, HMOs have the power to negotiate charges for many services. Furthermore, pre-approval requirements enable HMO insurers to control access to services and to deny payments for treatments they deem excessive or unnecessary, thus effectively removing both the patient and the doctor from the decision-making process and making health-care rationing a startling new reality.

Another side effect of HMOs was an increase in medical malpractice litigation, based on lack of treatment, poor treatment, and failure to accurately diagnose. The cost of malpractice insurance became a major factor in the cost of medical care in general. Once again, a system in which neither doctor nor patient "wins" took on a major role in driving America's massive health-care industry. And more than ever, distrust on both sides permeated the doctor–patient relationship.

FREE MEDS TO THE DOCTORS

The 1970s ushered in growing suspicions among the general populace about the industry's motives in the delivery of general health care. In the early part of that decade our economy wasn't doing well, even as health-care costs and physician salaries continued their rapid climb. Word leaked that some pharmaceutical companies plied doctors not only with more than 2 billion drug samples, but also with gifts in return for prescribing their drugs, a practice viewed by many as little more than bribery and casting doubts upon how motivated doctors were by patient well-being when it came to prescribing drugs. Physicians are human, after all, and not immune to the lure of advertising and freebies." In 1973, a survey revealed that 20 pharmaceutical companies gave away more than 12 million gifts, 45 million note pads, pens, and other "reminder items" logoed with the company's or its product's name, and all-expenses-paid cruises or trips to special "conferences" in resort locations. Medical suppliers eagerly joined in the process, too, offering physicians gifts as an encouragement to prescribe use of their equipment in treatment programs.

The upshot was that the relationship between patients and doctors and the health-care industry underwent a significant shift. For many Americans, the 1970s also were the beginning of the end of the era of the venerable, trusted family doctor and the onset of our experience as hapless (and often disgruntled) pawns in the big business of medicine. Although the practice of "fee-splitting," or sharing fees with a referring physician, had long been banned by the AMA, we began wondering about the legitimacy of physician referrals and hospital commitments. How did we know that our doctors weren't getting kickbacks for sending us to specialists, ordering certain tests, or admitting us to specific hospitals for treatment? According to their code of ethics, doctors were not allowed to compete with each other in pricing, and as members of a "learned profession," they were exempted by the courts from anti-trust laws. Most patients were, therefore, barred from comparing costs or quality of service among multiple health-care services.

Effectively, doctors could write their own ticket when it came to setting fees, and their salaries reflected that freedom. In a study published in 1978 by the Council on Wage and Price Stability, researchers found that between 1950 and 1977, physician fees and salaries outpaced salary inflation in other professions by over 43 percent. So as we paid more and more in medical fees, and as insurance costs climbed right along with government expenditures on health care, doctors, along with the rest of the medical industry, prospered greatly. And the economic and social divide between average Americans and their caregivers grew even wider.

In 2002, in response to growing public dissatisfaction with the cozy relationship between doctors and drug manufacturers, the drug industry put a new code in place that prohibited some of the most egregious giveaways, including expensive golf and vacation outings, dinners, and tickets to athletic events. Pharmaceutical companies responded by offering catered lunches during drug pitches and other perks that flew under the radar of the new codes. With a multi-billion-dollar industry at stake, these companies weren't going to walk away from practices that had served them so well in the past. Meanwhile, all of us in America were left wondering who held the allegiance of our doctors — we patients, or the suppliers to the industry?

Chapter 3
Shop for a Doc

ABOVE ALL, BEING a wise medical consumer means choosing medical partners we can communicate with effectively and trust. When it comes to protecting our health, we have to be sure that we are getting what we pay for. An engaged, concerned, and skilled doctor is the best health-care investment we can hope to find.

Let's Talk

Toward that goal, perhaps the most important step to becoming a smart medical consumer is the process of finding and choosing the right GP or family physician. That person will be your closest medical partner and will play an important role in helping you make other decisions about your health-care management and practitioners. If you are in the market for a new physician, ask your friends and coworkers for recommendations, and go online to find out what doctors within that specialty are located in your area. When you've found one you want to "interview," call the office and schedule an introductory appointment, so you can go in, share your medical history, and get a sense of the doctor's attitudes and approach to medicine (be sure to tell the scheduling assistant specifically what you want to do in the appointment so it is scheduled to give you adequate time).

As with any interview, little things count: the office workers, nurses, and med techs should be friendly and helpful; the office should be clean; the doctor should be open and willing to talk with you about your concerns and interests. Keep it relatively simple — no doctor will have hours to sit and chat. But use your time to determine how well this physician's working approach suits your own. Does he or she communicate with patients via e-mail, when appropriate? Is this doctor comfortable discussing information you've gathered? What hospital affiliations does the practice maintain? What regular screening tests does he recommend for someone of your age group, and on what schedule? Talk about your major health concerns and listen closely to the answers you receive. If you're comfortable with the initial meeting, schedule a full physical for another visit, and use that experience to cement or break the deal with this doc.

For the initial interview process I have developed a set of questions that I believe are important:

- How long have you been practicing?
- Where did you go to school, and where did you train? (It would be nice to know their class ranking but it's a bit tricky and may not be relevant.)
- Why did you choose this specialty or field of medicine?
- Have you ever been put on probation by the state medical board? If so, for what reason?
- Why did you become a doctor?
- How do you keep up to date with new information on treatments and research?
- Do you rely on pharmaceutical companies to provide your updates on the latest treatments?
- Do you have a physician assistant? How would I expect to interact with her/him?
- How many procedures like mine have you done?
- What is the most important thing about you that I should know?

BECOME A PARTNER WITH YOUR PHYSICIAN

Doctors are not infallible, nor should we expect them to be. Like the rest of us, they occasionally will be distracted and disengaged, and they won't always seek our active collaboration in the doctor-patient relationship. It is therefore our responsibility to speak up, ask questions, and insist that our voices are heard when we have concerns about our treatment.

We don't need a degree in medicine to partner with our doctors. We can start with some very simple steps. First, we should realize that our medical history is our business, not just our doctors' "property." Most of us know that we should maintain a list of our medications, including dosages and directions for use. In addition, many patient advocates today advise that we keep track of our medical records, requesting copies from our doctors for our own safekeeping. That way, we know exactly what information is available to new physicians and consulting specialists — and we have the important information we need if we want to do our own research into our symptoms, conditions, or treatment plans. Further, with copies of our test results in hand, we can be sure that the correct name appears on them and that there wasn't a mix-up at the lab.

BE YOUR OWN RECORDS-KEEPER

Every time you visit a new doctor, you're asked to complete a personal health information form that lists family medical history, your history of diseases, illnesses, injuries, hospitalizations, allergies, and so on. You're also asked to complete a "release of information" form, which enables your previous doctor to release health records to the new doctor's office. With all of this information floating around, you might wonder why anyone would need to keep his or her own personal health record. But, according to the American Health Information Management Association (AHIMA), *everyone* should do so. That way, no matter when or where we need health care, the medical provider we consult has access to a full and detailed medical history. There's a good chance that within the next several years this kind of database will be created and maintained by a central medical authority; but until then, we can and should keep our own medical records on file.

Your personal records might contain information your regular doctor might not record, such as your diet or exercise program, or your progress toward specific fitness goals. If you become ill or injured while traveling, during a move to a new city, during a local or national emergency, or anytime your regular physician's office is closed, access to your personal health records can be a valuable asset to anyone evaluating or treating your condition.

These records can be in written or electronic form, stored in a file folder, on a computer hard drive or disk, on a portable USB removable flash drive, or through an online service. The AHIMA maintains a web site (My Personal Health Record, at http://www.myphr.com) that offers full information about the benefits of maintaining a personal health record, along with electronic forms for compiling one and a search feature to find forms, tools, software, and services for storing your records. Online services typically have access codes and other measures devised to keep your information secure and accessible only by those you've authorized. Some online storage services are free, while others charge a monthly fee; if you're interested in online storage for your records, check each service carefully when making your choice. Keeping accurate and complete records takes time and effort, but it's our insurance that every doctor we see has access to the full story of our medical history.

WHAT IS A MEDICAL ADVOCATE?

At some point, most of us will need a medical advocate — a friend or relative who can accompany us to our appointment or examination to help take notes, ask questions, and listen to information. If our doctor wants to send us on our way with a prescription, we first should ask for the drug's name, its purpose, side effects, potential negative interactions, and so on. Then, when we fill the prescription, we need to check its accuracy before we leave the pharmacy. And we should always feel free to ask "why": Why do I need this drug, treatment, or surgery? How else could we tackle this problem? What benefits will I get from this treatment plan, and what risks am I taking?

It's also important to remember that doctors are just as prone to stereotyping as we are. If we suspect that a doctor's diagnosis might be influenced by his or her assessment of our (or our family member's) personality, sex, general appearance, or other first-glance attributes, or if we think the doctor might be categorizing us based only on a few obvious symptoms, we have every right to probe the reasons behind the diagnosis.

Doctors can be prickly, however, when they sense that their authority is being challenged. So how do we help make sure that our physician isn't misdiagnosing our condition? Jerome Groopman, MD, recommends that patients or their advocates describe to their doctors exactly what worries them the most about their symptoms or condition. And ask early — don't leave important details until the doctor is leaving the room. Groopman also suggests that patients ask questions to make their doctors think more deeply about their diagnosis, such as, "What else could this be?" or, "Could two things be going on at the same time?"

We shouldn't hesitate to speak up about sloppy practices, either. If our doctor forgets to wash her hands, or our nurse fails to notice that our IV has become loose, we'll be the ones who might suffer from a resulting infection. We can — and need to — ask whether all medical instruments, including stethoscopes and blood-pressure armbands, have been sterilized, and whether we should be started on antibiotics *before* surgery, to help ward off post-surgical infections. Whenever something about our care just doesn't seem right, we need to ask for an explanation *before* we continue with the plan.

Today, most doctors' offices send a packet of forms to new patients for the sake of providing your health and medical background. If you are developing your own computer-generated medical history, these forms would be helpful to see the kind of information doctors need to know. Be sure to include any alternative health practices and supplements.

Withhold nothing about your medical history, even if your unhealthy past may be embarrassing due to drugs, alcohol, sexual diseases or poor health habits. Doing so will only make it more difficult to get an accurate diagnosis, and may even lead to misdiagnosis. Keep in mind that there is probably nothing shocking to a doctor, and mind-reading is not one of the skills taught in medical schools.

Try to imagine a reversal of roles, with you as the doctor looking at yourself. Medical training will have taught you to study everything about how you look and act, including the color and condition of your skin and eyes, your energy level, and demeanor. This first glance tells a lot about your general health. What can't be determined is "the inside story." That's when a variety of tests may be ordered, such as a blood analysis, X-rays, and other diagnostics.

PATIENT–PHYSICIAN COMPATIBILITY OR NOT?

Through the years, my expectations for physicians have changed. If I'm going to need ongoing service, such as from a cardiologist, dermatologist, internist, or gynecologist, then compatibility is much more important. I remember a first encounter with a new-to-me internist who, by the end of the appointment, had managed to convince me that he had very little interest in me or my outcome. Apparently, this attitude permeated the office because his assistant did not bother to contact me to schedule a suggested test. The doctor seemed to feel no loyalty to me, and I certainly didn't feel any toward him. This kind of encounter means that it is time to move on.

On the other hand, if you're seeing a specialist for a (hopefully) one-time treatment, such as an oncologist or surgeon, personality is not as important. What you really want to know is, "How good is the doctor for this type of medical treatment?" A good question to ask in the first meeting is, "What is your success rate?"

One of my most recent medical experiences is a perfect example of the difference between using known and new doctors — and being an active participant in a treatment plan. I was being examined by my dermatologist for my annual "mole check." During the examination, I mentioned an unusual itch on my vulva. (It had been there at my previous visit but I didn't think it was important so I didn't mention it.) Immediately, she said, "This needs a biopsy."

One week later, she called to tell me that I have a very rare condition — extramammary Paget's disease — which is most often found in postmenopausal white women, and which causes a precancerous small growth in the vaginal area.

My next stop was my gynecologist, who had been notified and further explained the problem. She recommended a gynecological oncologist for surgical removal of the growth. She told me that this was the only surgeon she wanted to use and that she, too, would be in the operating room to protect me, her patient. I found this to be very comforting because I knew and trusted her, but I didn't know the surgeon.

The surgery was performed and a biopsy was done on the removed growth. The surgeon's recommendation was that I have a second, much more radical surgery to remove more tissue from the original area and to remove lymph nodes from both sides of the groin area to eliminate any cancer cells that might have spread further.

I felt I needed to have additional consultations since the disease was so rare. Through a friend who worked at the cancer center at a nearby medical school, I obtained the name of another gynecological oncologist. (There are only nine of these specialists in our entire state.) My original doctor was young, probably no more than thirty-five, and was following a very conservative approach. The second doctor was older — perhaps about fifty — and much more experienced. He explained everything he knew about the disease and my diagnosis/prognosis. After a long discussion, I decided that I would not have the second surgery. (I also talked with a third doctor since there was a difference of opinion.)

When patients make a decision, they also need to take full responsibility for it and the outcome. I scheduled a follow-up visit with my original oncologist and told him my decision. We then decided on a course of treatment that involves an examination every two to three months. Because Paget's is a disease, there is a strong possibility that there will be additional growths. Now, though, I know the only symptom (an itch in one spot) and will probably never need surgery as extensive as the first one.

Shop for a Doc

I firmly believe it's important for patients to be accountable for their bodies and health. We are in a professional relationship with our physicians. We may form close bonds with the health-care teams that tend to us or our loved ones, but we can't afford to overlook potential warning signs simply because we like and trust them. Mistakes happen all the time. Better that we ask why an order has been changed, why a vital sign has altered, why a medication has been dropped or started, than that a simple slip-up goes unchecked and develops into a fatal medical error.

CHAPTER 4
BEWARE OF DOCTOR GOD

"ANYONE WHO'S CONSIDERING this should be prepared to give up control of their life," a medical student told me when describing what she and others like her face when they set out to become doctors. "For at least seven years, and more like ten, you won't have control of your time — not your days or nights, when you will get home in the evening, when you can take a vacation, whether you can be in a wedding. You can't make plans for *anything* more than two weeks in advance. Your life is going to be taken out of your hands for almost ten years, and if you can't deal with that, don't enter the field."

I appreciated the young woman's graciously taking the time to talk about the rigors of her training. I never realized or considered these issues when on the sofa watching heart-warming medical dramas such as *Doctor Kildare*, *Ben Casey*, and of course, good old *Marcus Welby, M.D.*

WHO AND WHY?

As patients, we want our doctors to be like the old-fashioned, compassionate docs on TV, to demonstrate more understanding and to connect more closely with our humanity, not just our medical conditions. But how well do we understand *them*? Many of the "truths" we've always accepted about doctors no longer apply; in fact, we know much less than we realize about what it means to be a doctor today. The grueling process of their education alone surely must have an impact on how they turn out.

Beware of Doctor God

Of course, many of us feel that we know quite a lot about doctors, based in part on our experience as well as cultural stereotypes and common wisdom, and much of that shared data tends to paint them in an unflattering light. Ask your friends sometime what they think about doctors. Sure, some people enjoy good relationships with their physicians, but often you're likely to hear that they are narcissistic, egotistical, arrogant, cold, emotionally detached, money-grubbing, and more devoted to protecting members of their profession than to caring for patients — or some variation on those themes. In short, they know a "Doctor God."

Like any stereotype, Doctor God is really an extreme caricature that bears little resemblance to most physicians; but still we cling to it. However, our preconceived notions about doctors actually hurt *us* by limiting our ability to work effectively with them and to rationally and fairly assess the quality of the treatment they provide. Preconceptions also have a negative impact on physicians and the medical profession in general. When society ceases to respect and support that profession, we drive away the people who are drawn to the field out of a motivation to help and serve others — the "good doctors" we so desperately need.

Untangling the facts hidden within accepted presumptions can be a difficult process, but it's an essential step in limiting their power. If doctors truly *do* share some common traits or characteristics, what is the source? Does medicine attract people with specific personality types? Are the flaws we see in doctors simply the unavoidable products of their training and work environment? Are patients, with our negative attitudes, suspicions, and resentments, contributing to or even *creating* some of the problems we experience with doctors?

Beyond the title and degree, what shared links of background, personality, strengths, and weaknesses connect the men and women who choose a career in medicine? Researchers have explored the answers to these questions for more than sixty years.

Of course, we don't require a scholarly study to outline the many problems of modern life — the stress of time demands, career pressures, conflicting responsibilities, self-doubt, alienation, and feelings of isolation. These all-too-common challenges of modern life can make maintaining a positive, well-balanced attitude difficult for anyone. As it turns out, however, doctors may be more vulnerable to some of these stressors than the rest of us.

To understand this increased vulnerability, consider three critical influences that studies have shown can contribute to psychological problems in doctors: the interests and personality traits typical among those drawn to medicine; the unique pressures and responsibilities of medical practice; and the importance of public perception to a doctor's success. In combination, these factors not only fuel emotional problems in some doctors, they also can make it more difficult for them to cope with those problems effectively or to find outside help in doing so.

No, doctors aren't "all alike," but over the years, psychologists have identified a number of personality traits and psychological characteristics shared by many medical students and practicing physicians. In 2001, the Royal Australian College of General Practitioners published a study on doctors' troubled marriages, citing findings from the early 1970s that indicated physicians were predisposed to obsessive personality characteristics, including self-doubt, guilt, excessive fear of failure or making a mistake, and an exaggerated sense of responsibility.

Another thirty-year study of physicians' psychological vulnerabilities, begun in 1972, found that they were more likely to demonstrate characteristics such as dependency, pessimism, and self-doubt. At follow-up, these doctors were more likely than their fellow non-physician subjects of the same socioeconomic level to experience problems in their marriages and alcohol and substance abuse.

These and other studies paint a picture of doctors as being highly competitive perfectionists who are extremely self-critical, unforgiving of errors, and unwilling to accept the limitations of their human frailties. In a 2000 edition of the *Southern Medical Journal*, researchers from East Tennessee State University cited studies indicating that doctors are especially unforgiving of themselves for making clinical errors. Traits such as perfectionism and self-doubt can be made worse by the macho, competitive cultures of medical training and practice — and they can be especially damaging to self-esteem and emotional health. Even though doctors know that mistakes are inevitable, they often feel they can't admit to their peers that they have made mistakes, and they expect little support from colleagues when errors *do* occur.

Given these realities, many physicians who become depressed, angry, exhausted or ill, or whose careers or marriages start to fall apart, condition themselves to simply ignore the problems and "keep going." This self-neglect is another physician characteristic cited by many sources. As the authors of the *Southern Medical Journal* study stated, physicians' "personal problems can be perceived as professional failings." This denial of physical and emotional needs and responses to life, not only sets the stage for the above-mentioned problems, it can even lead to suicide.

But are doctors narcissists? Patients have talked about this subject for years, as have a number of research groups. To enter the discussion, it's important to understand the difference between full-blown, diagnosable narcissistic personality disorder (NPD) and narcissistic personality traits. In other words, a person might act like a narcissist without really *being* one; the difference is important.

True NPD is a severe disorder that, according to most estimates, affects less than 1 percent of the general population. Those with NPD have an exaggerated sense of personal importance, lack empathy, possess fragile self-esteem, and demand constant appreciation and praise from others in order to function. If they feel inadequately appreciated or if their behavior is questioned in any way, true narcissists are likely to lash out in anger or withdraw completely; they simply aren't able to cope with the normal, day-to-day demands of the world around them. They are psychologically unhealthy and, therefore, rarely have healthy relationships.

On the other hand, people who simply have narcissistic personality traits or behavior styles might be perfectly healthy psychologically, despite displaying a number of annoying (even unbearable) characteristics. This group tends to be arrogant and overly confident, prone to boasting, frequently guilty of ignoring the ideas and opinions of others, and dismissive of anything that doesn't reflect or involve their own interests. As overbearing or unpleasant as these individuals may be, they're healthier than those diagnosed with true NPD, because they aren't pathologically dependent upon the acceptance, admiration, and praise of others. Nevertheless, their behavior can be destructive to professional and personal relationships.

The medical profession has attracted both types of individuals; it may even have helped to create a few of them. John Banja, Assistant Director for Health Sciences and Clinical Ethics and Associate Professor of Clinical Ethics at Emory University School of Medicine, wrote extensively on the topic of narcissistic doctors in his book *Medical Errors and Medical Narcissism*. In an interview, Banja described the type of narcissist he encounters most frequently in medicine (who may or may not be diagnosed as having true NPD) as being someone who is "very bright, compulsive, hard-working," but who has lost his or her ability to be empathetic. To adapt to a stressful and demanding environment, an individual with narcissistic personality traits develops coping skills that basically block out everyone else.

"This is a person," says Banja, "who has forgotten how to monitor his or her relational skills."

Rather than "nature," Banja believes that "nurture" — in both the physician's upbringing and medical training — feeds narcissistic personality styles by teaching doctors-to-be that they are wonderful, special people, and that they must at all times appear to be infallible. Medical narcissists are loath to admit to any hesitancy or uncertainty, and they certainly don't want to ever admit that they are wrong. Medical narcissism, therefore, can play an especially damaging role in the aftermath of medical errors.

Although narcissistic traits aren't limited to male physicians, males seem to occupy center stage in both the published reports and most of the first-person accounts of medical narcissism described by people we interviewed for this book. Many of these sources offer the same description of the narcissistic physician's childhood and early development:

- A child who received uneven attention, who was either treated like royalty or neglected emotionally.
- A young person who decided to enter medicine as a way of cementing the idea of his or her special status, whose choice of specialty was guided largely by its promise of prestige, power, and monetary reward.
- A person driven by an extreme fear of failure, who may be devoted to either profession or family, but who simply cannot endure any kind of perceived threat to his or her omnipotence; these doctors can be emotionally abusive to their patients, coworkers, and families.
- A physician who is envious and fearful of colleagues, who strives relentlessly to win professional respect and recognition, and who can react with explosive rage or emotional collapse when confronted with any suggestion of error or omission.
- A spouse who is detached from many elements of his or her family life, but who demands complete control over others; a parent who is quick to criticize.
- A troubled individual at risk for abusing alcohol or drugs, and who might indulge in other risk-taking and self-destructive behavior.

Of course, the elements of narcissistic behavior aren't limited to doctors. In *The Medical Marriage*, clinical psychologists Wayne and Mary Sotile state their belief that most intelligent, driven people in high-performance careers eventually become "mature narcissists" in order to cope with the complex lives they lead. The Sotiles posit that this kind of narcissism isn't necessarily bad for individuals or their relationships — in fact, they believe that a certain degree of self-focus and egotism is probably just an adaptation to a demanding life. But they also note research suggesting that the same personality traits prompting people to become doctors can also contribute to the type of narcissism that can "propel them into lives filled with excessive work, trouble in intimate relationships, emotional struggle, poor self-care, and susceptibility to substance abuse and depression."

WHAT DOES MED SCHOOL HAVE TO DO WITH PERSONALITY?

Doctors who completed medical school before 1985 found themselves working in an unfamiliar environment in the last part of the century as they faced managed care, insurance oversight, hospital and clinic employers, team medicine, consumer-driven medical care, and the ever-present threat of malpractice litigation. Like personal computers, these facts of medical life today were practically unheard of until the mid-1980s. Those of us on the other side of the stethoscope have had to adjust to the same changing realities. Anyone over the age of forty has learned to be comfortable within the new doctor–patient relationship and changing medical environment. Younger doctors and their patients, meanwhile, struggle to overcome problems within a seemingly deeply flawed system.

Of course, medical schools also have undergone significant changes during the past few decades. Many today require that students take courses specifically addressing how to better provide compassionate and coordinated care within large practices and impersonal medical facilities. Licensing and accreditation boards responded to the public's clamor for fewer medical mistakes and more engaged and caring physicians by changing the way hospitals train interns and residents.

The medical community is changing from the inside, too. Open the doors of most medical school classrooms, and you'll observe a very different group of students than you would have seen twenty years ago. Many other professions today offer higher salaries, better working hours, fewer demands, and less stress than the practice of medicine. The once-coveted MD degree is no longer as attractive as it once was to people whose career choice is primarily motivated by a desire for money, prestige, and power. Furthermore, today's med-school graduates include ever-growing percentages of women and minorities.

Many of the changes in American medicine are reflected in the process of becoming a doctor. From getting into med school to surviving residency, what experiences and demands do doctors-to-be encounter on their path to entering a full practice? How are medical schools training them to cope with the realities of practicing medicine in modern-day America, and what kinds of doctors can we expect to emerge from that training? Will the "feminization" of medicine result in more engaged and compassionate doctors, or will America find itself with a shortage of high-level medical specialists and experienced GPs?

In 1991, Robert Marion, who was then Associate Professor of Pediatrics and member of the Admissions Committee at the Albert Einstein College of Medicine in New York, published *Learning to Play God*, his second groundbreaking work about the life of medical students in training. In the book's prologue Marion wrote that when he asked med-school applicants to explain their decision to become a doctor, well over 90 percent responded that they wanted to help drive scientific advancement and use their lives to help others. While Marion believed that this humanitarian desire is critical for anyone seeking a career in medicine, he also questioned whether the medical training system around the United States at that time was capable of sustaining — let alone nurturing — those best instincts of incoming medical students.

In the 1990s, Marion was not alone in his concerns about the effectiveness and safety of traditional medical training programs. For almost one hundred years, medical students worked continuous shifts of 100 to 120 hours, snatching a few hours of sleep at the hospital when possible. Residents, even interns, were often left to manage emergency room admissions and critical care patients with little support from their supervising physicians. Today, even with stricter regulations controlling duty hours and supervision, residency is still tough. Few professional training programs demand the stamina, determination, intelligence, and commitment required of medical students in the United States.

Many people think the boot-camp-like hours and rigorous demands of residency are essential to the process of becoming a doctor, and most agree the experience contributes to the perception of doctors as superhuman. As one interviewee put it, "When you consider what these people have to go through in order to become a doctor — let alone the important life-and-death decisions some make on a daily basis — you can almost understand why they might feel superior to the average person."

In other words, most individuals with first-hand exposure to the demands of medical training agree that mastering the science of medicine takes a strong intellect, strong talent, *and* a strong ego. And those traits can make it more difficult for some doctors to learn the art of dealing effectively with other people.

Wherever one receives medical education, becoming a doctor is an enormous undertaking. Acceptance alone is a huge hurdle. Most medical schools require applicants to have a year each of both organic and inorganic chemistry, a year of biology, a year of calculus, and a superior overall undergraduate GPA. Even with the best grades, the best undergraduate coursework, and the best Medical College Admission Test (MCAT) scores, gaining entrance to medical school is difficult. Fewer than half of the students who apply are accepted, and getting into top-rated schools, such as Harvard, Johns Hopkins, and the University of Pennsylvania, is incredibly difficult. In 2004, Harvard's medical school admission rate was just under 3 percent.

Those who do gain admittance take on a four-year course of classroom and clinical training. The first two years typically include preclinical coursework in anatomy, biochemistry, molecular biology, genetics, neuroscience, physiology, microbiology, immunology, pathology, diagnosis, pharmacology, medical ethics, humanities, and other demanding subjects — no "fluff" courses here. At the end of the second year, students must pass the Step 1 portion of the United States Medical Licensing Exam (USMLE). During the third year, they finish the clinical portion of their training, completing eight-week rotations in internal medicine, pediatrics, surgery, obstetrics and gynecology, and other medical departments within the hospital. Fourth-year students also complete rotations, typically focusing on a chosen area of specialization. At the end of the fourth year, students take Step 2 of the USMLE; Step 3 is taken during their internship/residency.

Although the program sounds daunting, after a medical school accepts a student, the institution works hard to make sure that student succeeds. More than 95 percent of all medical school enrollees are awarded an MD degree. However, the degree carries a hefty price tag. According to the American Medical Student Association, nearly half of all medical students begin their careers with educational debt in excess of $150,000 and a "significant minority" report that their debt tops $350,000.

Most doctors agree that getting through medical school is the easiest part of the training process. After graduation, aspiring doctors must work full-time in a clinical setting to finish internship and residency requirements. Internship, the first post-graduate year of training, is almost always acknowledged as being the toughest year of residency, which can last from three to six years depending upon the area of specialization. Many doctors complete a post-residency fellowship for subspecialty training. Meanwhile, the pay scale isn't all that great: On average, residencies pay about $35,000 a year.

So what specifically do these new doctors do? Interns work rotations, gaining experience in a number of specialties or areas within a single specialty. In the course of rotations, they complete rounds, forming a team of other students and attending physicians who visit a series of individual patients in a hospital or clinic. The interns speak with the patients and listen to attending physicians as they discuss the patients' conditions, diagnoses, and suggested treatment options. As occupants of the lowest rung of the ladder in any teaching hospital, interns can expect the nastiest, dreariest, and least-fulfilling "scut work" that arises during their shift. By the end of that first year of residency, though, most interns have determined the area of medicine they want to specialize in, then target the remaining years of residency toward that goal.

The second year of residency encompasses a great deal more responsibility, with more patient interaction and greater weight in suggesting treatment options. Often, residents are responsible for assessing and examining newly admitted patients and ordering tests and medications as necessary. Emergency room and intensive care unit residencies require split-second decisions and critical care for multiple patients suffering from life-threatening illnesses or injuries. Learning takes place quickly and often on the run. "See one, do one, teach one" is the typical on-the-job training program for most residents. Because they are still completing their medical education, they're also expected to attend lectures and conferences, and to study medical literature. All residents have on-call shifts as well, with only one day in seven set aside for no medical training duties.

Robert Marion's first book, *The Intern Blues*, relates the harrowing stories of three interns training in teaching hospitals in the Bronx during the mid-1980s. First published in 1989, the book has become an underground classic; many reviewers consider it still to be one of the most insightful and realistic accounts of medical internships ever written. The interns whose audio-diaries supplied content for *The Intern Blues* worked under conditions considered the norm for medical training at that time: 120-hour workweeks; on-call shifts of 36 or more hours; and 18- to 24-hour stretches at one time spent in the emergency room.

By the time the book hit the shelves, however, New York had adopted groundbreaking regulations that dramatically changed working conditions for young doctors in training. In 1984, a young woman named Libby Zion died within eight hours of being admitted to New York Hospital. Her family brought a wrongful death suit, charging that the attending doctors had killed Ms. Zion through misdiagnosis and mistreatment. Publicity surrounding the case cast a harsh light on the inhumane and dangerous schedules for internship and residency duty hours and the sometimes lax attendance of supervising physicians. The ensuing Bell Commission Regulations in

New York limited interns to no more than eighty hours of work in any week, and twenty-four hours in any single shift, with no more than twelve hours spent in any single ER shift. In 2003, the Accreditation Council for Graduate Medical Education (ACGME — the group responsible for accrediting post-graduate medical training programs within the United States) issued similar guidelines for all medical residency programs.

But in September of 2006, the *Journal of the American Medical Association* (JAMA) issued a new report on the dangers of "marathon" shifts of twenty-four hours or longer for medical interns. The *JAMA* study authors found that sleep-deprived medical staff were 5 times more likely to make misdiagnoses and 61 percent more likely to injure themselves with needles and scalpels. In a similar study, researchers found that when interviewed confidentially, some interns reported that they were not following the new ACGME guidelines, working sixty to seventy consecutive hours at a time.

We asked one medical student how closely residents in her program followed the work-hour regulations.

"The regulations don't make much difference," she replied. "For me, working with surgery residents, it takes a lot of hours. Every single resident on that rotation lied about their duty hours, every single week; they all work over 100 hours a week, but they don't write it down."

In a 2001 preface to a new edition of *The Intern Blues*, after the Bell Commission regulations were in place, Marion included an interview with an intern who reported that the experience of internship was still "brutal," leaving her exhausted and frightened that she "was going to accidentally screw up and kill someone."

Still, many doctors and medical educators have expressed concerns about the potentially *negative* impact of the new residency duty-hours regulations. Shorter shifts result in more "hand-offs," as residents exiting their shift turn over patient care to incoming replacements, and some educators worry that patient care will lapse as a result.

"No one wants doctors-in-training to adopt a 'day shift' mentality when it comes to patient care," one doctor we interviewed said. "Doctors can't simply walk away from a medical procedure or emergency because their shift is over."

Other educators worry that residents working limited shifts can't truly learn how to diagnose and treat conditions when they can't observe those conditions as they fully unfold over time. In a 2005 interview for National Public Radio's Boston affiliate, WCFR, Ron Goodspeed, MD, reminded listeners that the term "resident" extends back to the traditional training practice that required learners to actually *live* at the hospital during their training. Like many medical educators, Goodspeed expressed the idea that long hours, because they allow a resident to follow a patient and his or her illness through the course of a hospital stay, are critical for the learning process. "If you're going to learn something as complex as medicine," Goodspeed explained, "you have to be here. You have to see it all."

In the epilogue of *The Intern Blues*, Marion wrote that the internship year of residency is when the student truly becomes a physician. "But in the process," he adds, "through the wearing down of the intern's spirit, that person also loses something he or she has carried, some innocence, some humanness, some fundamental respect." When Marion revisited the interns profiled in his book, some fifteen years after their residency experience, all but one of them reported that the pains of that experience were worth the benefits of their careers. However, many in medicine today are less satisfied with their chosen profession, and that dissatisfaction has become a major factor in the rift between doctors and patients and the declining quality of health care in our country. What can we do to create a system that produces more caring, humane doctors? In the course of our exploration/research, we discovered that in Indiana some educators are already addressing that issue.

PHYSICIAN COMPETENCIES ARE NOW REQUIRED

If most students enter medical school with a burning desire to serve humanity, at some point during their training many will find that desire dampened considerably. Even barring narcissism, some come out of residency battle-hardened and cynical, with attitudes that make it difficult for them to work effectively with patients and their families, as well as with other doctors, nurses, and other medical services personnel. Although a certain degree of disillusionment accompanies any first-time "real world" career experience, many medical schools are making an effort to help graduates retain the humanitarian drive that first drew them toward the profession. Indiana University School of Medicine — which has the nation's second-largest medical student body — is a leader in this effort. Today, IUSM attracts some of the nation's brightest medical students, and schools across the country are adopting its curriculum model.

Stephen Leapman, MD, is IUSM's former executive associate dean for educational affairs and Dolores and John Read Professor of Medical Education. Leapman was one of the principal designers of IUSM's Competency-based Curriculum, an approach the school has used since 2003 to train students to become caring, complete physicians. Leapman described the program and its success, and the students undertaking medical training today.

"We've seen many changes," he began, "but that's been nationwide, rather than just with the IU student body. If you look at matriculation data, across the country, it's almost a fifty-fifty split between men and women. Unquestionably, we're interested in enrolling students into this class who are diverse in their demographics."

Leapman reported that IUSM continues to enjoy growing enrollment numbers. "In fact," he noted, "two years ago we had a 25 percent increase in the number of students applying to our medical school; last year, we had a 5 percent or 6 percent increase. Both of those years saw a greater increase in applications here than was reported nationally."

What about all the surveys out there indicating that doctors are increasingly dissatisfied with their workplace that some analysts worry might be steering qualified candidates away from careers in medicine? Furthermore, we mentioned that some of the doctors interviewed for this book stated specifically that they had perceived a decline in both the quality and the work ethic of today's medical students. Leapman disagreed.

"At IU, we're finding the caliber of the student applying to our school is higher than ever. The GPA of admitted students entering our school this year was 3.73 overall, and the MCAT scores were the best we've ever seen. We're getting very high-caliber students. And even though we are seeing physicians retire earlier because of changes in the workplace, those changes aren't noticeable to students entering the profession today who don't recall what it was like fifteen or twenty years ago. They only see one end of the spectrum, and that's going to be a medical practice dominated by influences such as insurance companies, other practice plans, and associated workforce issues."

But the big story at IUSM is its competency-based curriculum, and what many refer to as its relationship-centered care initiative; this reflects a commitment to produce well-rounded physicians who excel at more than the clinical skills required of any doctor.

Leapman explained IU's decision to adopt the curriculum. "In the early '90s, there was a movement throughout the country to change the way we were training medical students. In Indiana, we felt that we had to go beyond simply teaching them what doctors are supposed to know — biochemistry, pediatrics, anatomy, and so on. All medical schools teach those courses, and all medical students are very bright and can learn from them. But nothing we were doing taught students the humanistic values that really make a physician complete. We looked around for a better curriculum and found one at Brown University — the competency-based curriculum. We embraced that and refined it; it's not perfect but we've exceeded what it was when we first encountered it.

"In that curriculum, we've defined nine competencies. Two of those are traditional physician competencies. The first is clinical skills — how you put in an intravenous line, how you put in a subtracheal line, how you interview a patient, and so on. And the other is how you use those clinical skills to correctly make diagnoses and to determine prognoses and management plans, using evidence-based medicine."

The other seven competencies Leapman described in detail:

- Communication skills: "We want our students to understand the necessary components of communication for physicians. We want them to know what informed consent really means, and we want them to be able to deliver bad news to a patient, to be understood by both the patient and family without being overbearing. And quite honestly, many physicians don't know how to do that."
- Lifelong learning: "Physicians have to be lifelong learners. Because of the amount of new information coming at doctors today, keeping up with developments in medicine is like trying to drink from a fire hose. So we teach our students how to judge the merits of what is coming out of the medical literature, because it's not all good."
- Self-awareness and personal growth: "When young men and women go to medical school, complete their residencies, and begin their practice, they can become overwhelmed. So when do they actually have time to sit back and reflect on who they are as a person, what they're doing, and what they're doing for their families? How do we teach self-awareness and personal growth? It may sound corny, but there's so much more to be learned from this work than which muscle connects to which bone. So much of medicine is humanity, and we want to unveil to our students the human nature of medicine."
- Social and community contexts of medicine: "This competency involves teaching students to relate to the society in which they practice medicine. We explore, for example, how practicing medicine on an Indian reservation in New Mexico differs from practicing medicine in downtown Gary, Indiana. This is an important understanding for doctors, particularly when our nation is becoming an even richer melting pot of cultures."
- Moral and ethical reasoning: IUSM considers this com-

petency to be absolutely critical for all of its students. The school has recently begun offering a combined MD and MA degree in philosophy and bioethics. The degree is too new to know exactly how students will apply it in the workplace, but Leapman is excited at the possibilities for this important new area of educational focus.

- Problem solving: This is at the heart of all good medical practice. As Leapman said, "The importance of that competency for physicians is pretty self-evident."
- Professionalism: Leapman described this as perhaps the most important competency taught in IUSM's curriculum. "We've spent an inordinate amount of time trying to make our students truly understand what's involved in being a professional practicing physician in the community."

IUSM expects all students to master these competencies and to treat them seriously, Leapman explained. "We make a lot of our admittance decisions on a holistic grid that looks not just at students' academics, but also at how they respond to our questions in regard to their attitudes toward these competencies. We've had some absolutely incredible, stellar individuals, who come from very good schools, and who academically are unbelievably talented, but who we determine, through our interview process, are absolute jerks. And we don't admit them to our medical school; that's not the kind of person we want to train to practice medicine."

Of course, IUSM isn't the only school today practicing a curriculum geared toward educating "the whole doctor." In 1999, the ACGME listed six core competencies for physician performance: patient care, medical knowledge, practice-based learning and improvement, system-based practice, professionalism, and interpersonal skills and communication. To be accredited in the United States today, every medical school must show positive proof that it presents and assesses these competencies in its program. "Therefore," as Leapman said, "competencies are becoming the buzzword of medical education."

Beware of Doctor God

Steve Leapman believes that public dissatisfaction with the medical status quo drove the movement toward competency-based training. "The populace of this country was tired of going to physicians who were so one-dimensional that they couldn't tell you anything other than how they were going to fix the ligament in your knee, and who cared more about your knee than they did about *you*.

"That's not what patients want," he continued. "If you ask patients what impresses them most about their physician, they aren't going to tell you that the doctor fixed their knee. To be honest, they expect that as a given. What they *want* is for you to be able to explain things to them, to be empathetic, to be there when they need you. That's what physicians since time immemorial have done, and that's what we have to reintroduce."

The importance of competency training for physicians goes beyond its benefits to patients, Leapman added. "Look at the malpractice data. Many of the suits that have been brought against physicians are really just the result of bad communication. If you establish a strong relationship with your patient, and you have a poor result — which is inevitable at some point — you're significantly less likely to be sued over that if you have rapport with your patient."

Leapman was also quick to point out the value of assessing medical students based on their level of competency in the skills taught at IUSM. "Maxine Papadakis, who is on the faculty of the University of California at San Francisco, has done studies of physicians who have lost their licenses in the state of California. After combing through their medical school records, she's discovered an incredible correlation between how medical students behave in school and the kind of decisions they'll make after they get their license. You know, in school, their supervisors record that a particular student might be smart, but maybe was lousy with patients." In other words, students who exhibit poor professionalism during medical school are likely to have professional problems later in medical practice.

In Leapman's medical school days, he said, no one was asked to leave for not behaving professionally or for poor communication skills. They were asked to leave because they had bad grades.

"Today," he said, "if you don't pass your competencies, you'll be asked to leave. When we first started this curriculum, we had a student who was a total jerk — he couldn't get along with anyone, he had a horrible attitude, he was terribly argumentative, and his evaluations for professionalism were in the toilet — and we dismissed him. One of our faculty members said, 'What are we doing here? I know this student and his family, this is a bright young guy, and we're dismissing him for this soft-fuzzy-feeling stuff. This is crazy!' This was an older faculty member who just didn't get it. It's not always an easy sell."

What about outcomes, though? Leapman assured us that the school has found plenty of data to show that the competency-based curriculum is working. IUSM students have a 99 percent pass rate for Step 1 of the USMLE exam, which is higher than the national rate, and they have a higher mean passing score. "So our students are doing significantly above the national average on these scores," Leapman noted. "Academically, they're doing just fine."

Leapman also pointed to data that indicate the students are happy with the core competency curriculum. "At the end of the year," he explained, "graduating seniors across the nation are asked to take the AAMC [Association of American Medical Colleges] graduation questionnaire. We don't administer this; it's a two- to three-hour survey of some sixteen thousand students. One of the questions asks if the student to rate his/her level of global satisfaction with his/her medical education. Prior to our initiation of the competency-based curriculum, the answer to that question from our students was not very high. In fact, we were below the national average.

"But," he continued, "with the class that matriculated in 2001, we began paying more attention to the students. We developed our core values and guiding principles to create a more user-friendly working and learning environment. Three years ago we met the national average for student satisfaction; two years ago, we were higher than the national average; last year we *far* exceeded the national average for students reporting that they liked the environment in which they learned medicine. We're pretty happy about that."

Not every student reports such heartfelt enthusiasm for the

school's curriculum when asked directly. A third-year medical student at IUSM assured us that she felt medical ethics are incredibly important and enjoys studying them, but she didn't think the "nontraditional" competencies taught at IUSM would have much impact on the way she and her classmates approach their work. "I think it's good that we have it," she said, "but I'm not sure that I feel it actually affects our day-to-day medical practice. In fact, most people I talk to think it's a waste of time." Some speculate that, in the male-dominated world of med school, acknowledging the value of training focused on building empathy, compassion, and understanding is considered a sign of weakness. But sometimes it takes an outsider's eye to really see the picture. When asked about her observations of the curriculum's impact on students, a librarian at IUSM's medical library responded with a chuckle. "When they first started the new curriculum, all of the students complained about it," she said. "Now, most of them love it."

Leapman believes that students *want* to master the skills at the center of IUSM's competency-based curriculum. "You know," he said, "I chaired our admissions committee. One question I always ask of students applying to our school from other states is, 'Why are you applying here?' The answer typically is, 'Because I went on the web and looked at all of the LCME-accredited [Liaison Committee on Medical Education] schools, and I was impressed with your competency-based curriculum. I know that you can make me a whole physician, and that's what I'm looking for.'"

Okay, so we all understand that medical training is rigorous, and we now know that it's changed a lot over the past few decades. Medical students are learning more social skills, working fewer hours (or at least they're *supposed* to be working fewer hours), and — in some specialties — expecting lower salaries than med school graduates did twenty years ago. Then what does all of this tell us about our own doctors and health-care experiences?

First, we should be aware that America's top medical schools understand the importance of communication and compassion in physician–patient relationships. That means we shouldn't feel like we're being overly needy if we insist that our doctors take the time to explain things thoroughly and to listen and respond to our concerns.

When we're being treated by interns or residents in a hospital or ER setting, we also need to remember that they may be suffering from fatigue due to long hours — in spite of work-hour regulations. The effects of that fatigue, which contributes to medical errors, have been compared to the effect of elevated blood-alcohol levels. All of this means that we absolutely *must* speak up when anything seems unusual or unnecessary about our treatment program. (That's true for any situation, but it's especially important when we're dealing with doctors or doctors-in-training who might be wrapping up thirty-six hours of nonstop work.) We don't have to be rude or confrontational to find out why we're having a certain test or taking a specific medication and what its effects will be. And we always have the right to ask for the attention of our attending physician.

It is also up to us to be aware of the potential for errors resulting from shift changes. If we're hospitalized or even in the emergency room for an extended period of time, we should try to find out when the shifts change and realize that incoming residents will be "getting up to speed" on our case. Again, we just need to speak up — or ask our attending physician — if we think they might have missed something important in the hand-off.

Finally, we really do need to remember that interns and residents are going through a grueling experience, and that we *want* them to get the best training possible. Even as we vigilantly monitor the treatment we get at the hands of doctors-to-be, we need to appreciate the hard, necessary work they're doing and treat them with the same respect we extend to any physician. After all, they're only human, not gods.

Not surprisingly, during residency, doctors can experience many problems associated with depression and exhaustion, including occasional thought impairment, chronic anger, cynicism, and break-downs in personal relationships. A 1975 study found rates of clinical depression among participating interns as high as 30 percent, with

25 percent reporting some suicidal thoughts. A more recent study at the University of California in San Francisco found that as many as *one-fourth* of the first- and second-year medical students at that school were depressed.

The negative effects of medical training can follow these individuals right along into their practices. While some doctors will try to ignore and "work through" their depression, others might attempt to self-medicate — a practice that can lead to substance abuse.

In *The Medical Marriage*, Wayne and Mary Sotile cite findings indicating that medical residents were five and one-half times more likely than the study's controls to use sleeping pills, stimulants, and other drugs. Other research has shown that, while doctors may be no more prone than others to abuse alcohol and illicit drugs, they might be more at risk for abusing prescription drugs — a problem that seems to escalate when residents are granted prescription-writing privileges.

Studies have reported conflicting findings about physician suicide, as well, but most experts agree that doctors have a higher incidence of suicide than those in the general population. In July of 2005, The American Foundation for Suicide Prevention cosponsored a summit on physician depression, specifically aimed at understanding the high rate of suicide among that group. An online report of that meeting stated that over 40 years of studies have shown that "on average, death by suicide is about 70 percent more likely among male physicians in the U.S. than among other professionals, and 250 to 400 percent higher among female physicians."

To put these statistics into perspective, think about this: Each year in the United States, 100 to 150 doctors commit suicide. That's like losing *every member* of a typical graduating class from a mid-size medical school in this country, *every year*.

Although startling to realize that male doctors are almost twice as likely to kill themselves as are nonphysician male professionals, the idea that female physicians have suicide rates two, three, or nearly *four* times greater than those outside the profession is truly sobering.

SICK OF DOCTORS?

We know that female doctors commit suicide much more often than do other women in our society, but we don't have much hard data as to *why* that's true. Most of the studies conducted on physician suicide are at least ten years old and focused firmly on white males. It's likely that this bias will change over the next few years because numerous sources have called for more research into the problem of female physician suicide. But for now, many psychologists, sociologists, and other experts depend on anecdotal evidence to explain this sad reality.

First, we know that female students may be more prone to suffer the effects of depression than their male counterparts. A study reported in 1990 found that nearly 40 percent of female and 27 percent of male medical students surveyed had experienced pronounced symptoms of depression or anxiety. That same study found that the rate of these symptoms reported by male students declined dramatically between medical school and residency, but female students didn't experience the same relief from their depression as they progressed through training. Some women in medicine, like their male counterparts, turn to drugs to help fight off fatigue, depression, and anxiety. Some studies have linked drug abuse in female doctors to the additional burden of their social role. Although drug abuse is certainly associated with suicide, current research doesn't provide a proven link between these problems and the high rates of suicide among female physicians.

Second, most sources agree that society expects a lot more from women in high-profile careers than it does from their male colleagues. Every female executive has felt the judgment of others descend on her as she carves out her own method for juggling the responsibilities of a demanding career with those of raising a family. The highly competitive environment of medicine only complicates the situation for women doctors. Establishing supportive close relationships within the profession can be difficult, leaving women to rely on their closest relationships outside work, and those relationships can be strained mightily by the demands of the medical profession.

Beware of Doctor God

As one medical student stated, "Most of the male surgery residents are married and have kids. None or few of the female residents have husbands and children. It's harder for women to do a residency with kids than it is for a male."

CHAPTER 5
QUESTION MOTIVES

WE, THE PATIENTS, really want to believe that our physician is 100 percent on our side, focused on us and with our health and well-being uppermost in his mind. But if you think about it for a minute, you have to wonder that if he or she has twenty-five patients scheduled for that day and we are allotted only fifteen minutes out of that, how "uppermost" can we be?

That is a dilemma all patients face. Further complicating the issue is that doctors, being human like the rest of us, have a life outside the clinic, and if that other part of their life is less than wonderful, it can affect their attitudes toward us. Thus, patients should indeed sometimes question their doctor's motives and recommendations.

When some ex-wives and nurses related their shocking life-with-physicians stories, I was not shocked because I had experienced some of what they told me first-hand, during my brief but nevertheless all-too-long marriage to one. The total life of a doctor *does* make a difference in his or her approach to patient care, more for some than for others.

Asking a physician questions about his or her personal life would be both difficult and inappropriate, but you can use other methods. For example, question prescriptions: what are they for, what is the dosage, and would another drug work just as effectively? Inquire about other recommendations for improving your health; if this irritates the doctor, that's a sure sign that you are not the center of his or her focus.

Remember, you are the customer who is responsible for seeing the doctor's bill is paid, and if necessary, you can fire him. Think about this as you read the following stories of dysfunctional docs.

BEHIND CLOSED DOORS — AT HOME . . .

"It's nobody's business what their doctor's life is like outside the office."

I heard that from a woman who had just gone through a divorce from her doctor husband of thirty-plus years. Why, she wondered, would anyone want to know about the personal lives of doctors? "I don't want to know about my attorney's private life!" she said with some exasperation.

That may be, but she wasn't getting the point of my queries. While it's true that doctors have no responsibility to bare their private lives to the general public, we can understand a great deal about how physicians deal with the outside world by learning more about how they function within family relationships.

Beyond the emergency room, surgical theater, or clinic office, these individuals are shaped by their personal relationships, and sometimes the "physician personality" takes a heavy hand in shaping those relationships as well.

Issues related to control, ego, image, and openness were often mentioned in the course of talking with doctors and those familiar with the challenges they face in their personal relationships. Personal problems stemming from such issues were more likely than not to be brushed off with comments such as, "Oh, yes, that's typical of doctors," or "Well, that's just what doctors are like."

"Many doctors have dysfunctional family lives," a psychologist remarked. "They tend to be controlling, detached, and needy of public approval, but disdainful of the emotional needs of their loved ones."

Needless to say, a doctor — or anyone, for that matter — who suffers from these kinds of emotional issues make lousy life partners. Fortunately, only a small percentage of doctors fall into this category. As tempting as it might be to believe that one's failed relationship with a physician is a victim of some sort of widespread Doctor God syndrome, learning the facts — and fallacies — that feed this negative perception of physicians and their ability to function on a personal level is more useful.

The troubled physician marriage has been the topic of a number of studies and publications. Psychiatrist Michael F. Myers outlined the marital issues he most frequently dealt with in his fifteen years of counseling physicians and their families in his book *Doctors' Marriages: A Look at the Problems and Their Solutions*. In male physician marriages, communication difficulties, overwork, alcohol abuse, self-medication, undiagnosed depression, sexual problems, and violence are major issue themes. In female physician marriages, guilt, poor self-image, role strain, and issues surrounding the husband's self-esteem and/or underemployment and feelings of belittlement add to this unhappy mix.

While many would agree the marital problems Myers describes appear not unusual, he and others who have studied these issues are careful to point out that, while these sources of marital difficulty aren't unique to doctors, doctors' marriages are especially vulnerable to them. In *The Medical Marriage*, Mary and Wayne Sotile note that many doctors pack a great deal of emotional baggage when they enter a marriage, often as a result of coming from families that offered little in the way of attention and nurturing. Any one of the personality traits associated with physicians, such as pessimism, perfectionism, and an overriding need to control, can threaten a strong and happy marriage; in combination, they can effectively kill a relationship.

As noted, the culture of medicine itself — from training to practice — can fuel the development of narcissism, depression, and substance abuse. When the physician marries, these vulnerabilities can infect the partnership, putting doctors' *spouses* at special risk for developing the same types of problems. Some spouses might identify so strongly with their physician partner or become so reliant on the prestige associated with medicine that they become self-absorbed or egotistical. Emotional neglect coupled with an unwillingness to admit to marital troubles can result in depression, alcoholism, and substance abuse for both partners in the marriage.

Question Motives

The experts are divided on the question of whether medical marriages suffer more problems leading to divorce than do non-medical marriages. The Sotiles' research indicates that physicians and their spouses suffer "significantly increased" incidences of drug abuse, alcoholism, depression, suicidal thoughts and acts, and psychiatric hospitalizations, as compared to those in the general population. In contrast, the April 1989 *Journal of the American Medical Association* published a report by Doherty and Burge noting that physicians actually have a *lower* tendency to divorce than do members of other occupational groups.

However, the data gets even more confusing. Some research indicates that the divorce rate for physicians varies dramatically, according to the doctor's gender and area of medical specialization. A 30-year study at Johns Hopkins, completed in 1997, showed an overall divorce rate of around 29 percent for American doctors; within areas of specialization the divorce rate varied between 22 and 51 percent. Furthermore, female physicians had a higher divorce rate (37 percent) than did their male colleagues.

Considering the overall U.S. divorce rate in 1997 was 43 percent, it appeared that most doctors then had more stable marriages than the average Joe or Joanne. That overall figure, however, included everyone, not just those within the physicians' socioeconomic group. Researchers caution, however, that just because a medical marriage remains intact doesn't necessarily mean it's happy or satisfying for either partner. As in other forms of self-neglect, some doctors and their spouses prefer to weather a troubled marriage rather than go through the emotional process of healing it or the financial and legal quagmire of ending it.

Perhaps a narcissistic focus on work may not necessarily be the *cause* of marital problems so much as one of the side effects. Most physicians are, by nature, hard-working, high-performance individuals; it's also true, though, that many of them find it easier to deal with the demands of their profession than to work on solving problems at home. When marital discord arises, these doctors are more likely to bury themselves in work, then react with wounded indignation when spouses call them on the carpet for investing too little time and attention in the marriage and family. "Hey," the thinking prevails, "that's what it's like to be married to a doctor, so you'll just have to get used to it."

Doctors' spouses also often appear to have difficulty addressing marital issues. They may face problems getting their spouse's attention or suffer from self-esteem issues. As in other high-profile, professional family households, the ties that bind troubled physician marriages may be woven out of necessity rather than love and mutual respect, and the spouses may be reluctant to rock the boat and risk further damage to a relationship upon which they feel socially and financially dependent.

However, physician marriages are changing beyond the traditional image of a male doctor with a stay-at-home wife. As more females enter medicine, doctor/doctor marriages are more common. According to a 1999 study published in the *Annals of Internal Medicine* (*AIM*), 22 percent of male and 44 percent of female physicians were married to members of their own profession. The report also indicated that a time is coming when half of all physician marriages in this country will be dual-doctor relationships. The dual-doctor marriage offers a great many benefits, including shared work experiences and interests and a greater family income. On the other hand, these benefits don't always extend to both partners.

In research published in 2002 by the Minnesota Medical Association, 65 percent of the women physicians surveyed reported that they performed more than half of all household chores, while their spouses contributed less time to that effort. In the 1999 *AIM* study mentioned above, 33 percent of female physicians in dual-doctor marriages reported "substantial limitations" in their professional lives, which they attributed to family obligations — limitations rarely reported by male physicians. Those women were more likely than their husbands (or their unmarried female colleagues) to interrupt their careers, and most of them noted that the time conflicts of a dual-doctor marriage are enormous. Even so, the divorce rate among those marriages was about standard to the general public.

Question Motives

When a marriage goes on the rocks, it can leave behind much bitterness and hurt feelings. A fractured physician marriage is no different. Some doctors' exes, however, remain almost protective of their defunct marriages, reluctant to talk about them — possibly a remnant of that fear of rocking the boat that induced the couple to stay together as long as they did.

"Audrey" was one whose advocacy for physicians spoke volumes about the degree to which she identified with her ex-husband's profession and about the impact her medical marriage had on her life. At first she was less than enthusiastic to share her story. She agreed to talk, then took it back. Finally, she consented — but only to a clearly stated point: "I don't want to answer questions that impinge on my private life," she said, evidently still misunderstanding the reason for the interview in the first place. Gradually she warmed more to the topic. Certainly, her story provides valuable insight.

Her ex-husband, "Ben," began college around 1950. Being Jewish, he faced the quota system that existed in those days and chose to go into medicine because he couldn't get into engineering school.

"That's an aspect of the medical profession you probably didn't think about," Audrey commented. "I mean, there were physicians who went into practice with other Jewish physicians or went into practice by themselves, and their patients would have been almost exclusively Jewish. That would be true today of a lot of minority physicians; probably not so much so, but it's still there. As a result, there are probably a lot of people who went into medicine who might have preferred to have done something else."

Audrey believed her cardiologist husband enjoyed the academic pursuit of medicine, which he found more interesting than the profession's other aspects. "He used medicine to pursue the kinds of inquiries that he was interested in," she said. "He attempted to influence his career choice, more than his career influenced him. He spent a lot of time doing research. He wrote a book. Most of his life was spent pursuing research topics and creating a name for himself."

Public recognition was important to Ben, but Audrey hesitated to say more about his personality or, for that matter, the "medical personality" type.

"I would say that people have a certain personality, no matter what they choose to do with their life," she said. "Their careers are molded by their personal goals and those can be accomplished with whatever career they choose. It wouldn't have mattered what career my husband chose, he would have pursued the same goals: to become an academic person and to further his reputation. Other aspects of his life would have been subservient to that.

"I don't know that he regretted his choice [to become a doctor] but I wouldn't say that he spent his life planning to be a physician or that achieving that goal satisfied his life's ambitions. His career was certainly the most important aspect of his life, though, I believe."

More important than his marriage? Audrey quickly defended Ben's focus on his career.

"Medicine requires a lot of energy. Most doctors of his generation were on call almost all the time — if not, it was because they chose a form of medicine that didn't require those hours of commitment. It takes a lot of energy and intellectual capacity to make it through medical school. Guys who are that driven and competent aren't going to waste time on what they consider to be frivolous activities."

She also numbered the other things that consumed so much of her husband's time, such as continuing education, preparation for new examinations, and licensing and certification processes to keep his credentials updated. "My husband had a lot of other talents," she conceded. "He was very athletic, played tennis, golf, racquetball. We used to travel a lot, he enjoyed that. He was a pretty busy guy."

She paused a moment in thought, then continued. "As the wife of a physician, you end up creating a life for yourself because you don't have a lot of time with your husband. If your husband is at all conscientious about his career, you just have to find your own life."

Still, Audrey enjoyed being a physician's wife, and even years after her divorce, she identifies deeply with the physician's perspective on life.

Question Motives

"Watching him and his colleagues who had different specialties, I observed people's ways of dealing with the career," she said. "The career is not a monolithic thing. Depending on where you practice, when you practice, and what you practice, your career can be very different. Many physicians have very different personalities, too."

Like the Doctor God stereotype?

Audrey clearly was ready for this question. "Okay, there are doctors that have a 'god' complex," she began. "Those are typically the surgeons or anyone who does something invasive as a specialty. Those are the people who generally have the most control over their careers and who have the greatest number of people dependent upon them, whether it's the people who work with them or the patients who rely on them. There are people who go into medicine because they want to be singled out from the general population in some way. They want to have some special category of definition, which they receive simply by being called 'Doctor' rather than 'Mister.' "

Did her ex conform to the stereotypes many people hold about doctors? Audrey wasn't sure. "People made the assumption that he was very wealthy, that he was very smart, that he was very busy. I don't know what people's assumptions are about doctors in terms of their caring qualities. I suppose, in a sense, they think that anyone who goes into medicine must care about people."

Were these assumptions accurate? "In terms of the financial aspect, probably not," she replied. "Physicians earn different levels of income, depending upon their specialty," she said. "My husband's income wasn't the same as a heart surgeon. Pediatricians don't earn as much as cardiologists, either. Still, physicians are in the top 1 percent of the population in terms of income, but within that 1 percent, there are people earning a lot more money than doctors. And many careers are a lot more financially rewarding than medicine. As far as being busy, most physicians are. And you can't get through medical school if you aren't extremely intelligent.

"In terms of caring about patients," she continued, "that varies with the person. It isn't necessarily a quality of all physicians."

Audrey seemed less certain about assumptions made about her

as a doctor's wife. She thought people who didn't know her probably had inflated assumptions, but not her friends. "We saw each other as individuals, not as our husband's wives. We were quite different, with different personalities. Most of us were married young, before we knew what our lives would be like as physicians' wives. I've never expected people to judge me on that basis. A lot of my friends weren't married to doctors, so that wasn't important to me.

"I'm a bright person; I went to a good college; I have a lot of interests, and I'm a very productive person. I didn't depend on my husband to create an identity for me. I can't speak for others, but that's my sense of myself.

"I know a lot of wives of successful men who pretty much cater to their husbands rather than having lives of their own. Many wives feel that if they're married to a high-performance individual, their role in life is to support that person. Others aren't willing to live simply to support their spouse's needs. Given a certain number of hours in the day, you either fill your time with a career or something else. In that respect, wives have to find something to fill their days. There are women married to physicians who aren't involved in activities of their own, but spend their time at home cooking and cleaning and waiting for their husbands to come home. Others go into the office and help their husbands at work. I don't think that many people realize what their lives will be like. My father wasn't a physician, so I didn't know what it would be like. Other women had doctor fathers, so they knew what they were getting into."

Audrey didn't think any of this had any relevance to narcissistic traits in doctors per se. "I might choose to say that my [ex]husband is a narcissist, but I don't think that's pertinent to his career as a physician. It's more pertinent to his relationship with his family. I certainly would not sit here and tell you that I think all physicians are narcissists. I know many women who are married to physicians who aren't narcissists, and I know many who are."

Audrey saw little purpose in exploring the topic of a doctor's life outside of work. She seemed surprised that people wouldn't already understand what it's like to be a doctor, and to support the notion that we should view our doctors from a respectful distance.

"Sharon" had a brief but nightmarish medical marriage that not only left her self-esteem battered and bruised, but offered her essentially little if anything in the way of prestige. She is a registered nurse who has worked in hospital settings for nearly thirty years. Over time, Sharon came to understand that she and her husband shared more than a profession in medicine: both suffered from addictions.

Their problems eventually overwhelmed the marriage, and the two divorced after four years. While together, Sharon came face to face with some ugly truths about her husband, herself, and the life they created.

Sharon graduated college with a bachelor of science in medicine (BSM), which has offered her a degree of career flexibility that she has enjoyed tremendously: risk management, medical legal review for malpractice cases, quality assurance, and work for insurance companies, as well as working in a clinical setting.

Like many other nurses, she met her husband, an ER physician, when she was working in that department of a large Indianapolis hospital. They knew each other several years before they even began dating, and she knew he was divorced and had custody of his child. She was forty-six years old and he forty-two when they married, old enough and experienced enough, one would think, to be able to make a good choice in a spouse. But soon, Sharon encountered one unpleasant surprise after another. Her husband's sensitivity skills, for example, left much to be desired — a trait she spotted early on.

"As a physician, his clinical skills were good," Sharon said. "As far as giving empathy or sympathy — no way. I've often wondered why he went into the field. I mean some doctors aren't capable of showing compassion, but they have it. I've never seen compassion in this man. I've heard him deliver bad news to people with a completely blank face and a canned 'I'm sorry for your loss.'

"He grew up in a large family and was very isolated. He was very,

very bright, but had no social skills. He was the oldest of twelve; seven were born to the family, five were adopted, and then there were a bunch of foster kids running through the house. He was the odd man out. He stayed apart from the others, he didn't like what they ate for supper, didn't like this, didn't like that. He was always pretty much isolated. His dad actually gave him a book that told him how to talk to people, ask them about themselves, shake hands, and so on. But nothing ever taught him how to deliver those pat phrases with any feeling. I've always wondered if maybe he had a personality disorder from the get-go."

Medicine was not Sharon's husband's first choice of careers. "He originally was going to go into psychology, because his father was a psychologist. He and my ex-husband's mother have written several books on child-rearing. I don't know whether sometimes his parents were off doing their thing and there was a break in the relationship or what. But with twelve kids and a bunch of foster kids, how can you ever give every kid everything they need? The kids took care of themselves; it's an interesting dynamic."

Sharon wasn't prepared for what was waiting for her after the "I dos" were exchanged. Her husband's behavior toward her switched dramatically — the Dr. Jekyll/Mr. Hyde phenomenon reported in some physician marriages. "We both had issues, of course," she admitted. "I think I carried my own Doctor God complex. I'd look at him and think 'oh my goodness, he's just so . . . so . . . yada-yada-yada.' I'd lost a lot of my self-esteem by then, too.

"But the day we got married, he totally freaked out. He became upset, almost angry at all of us. He became so critical and withdrawn that I took my luggage out of the car and said, 'I'm not doing this!' Then we talked it through and went ahead and got married. I've since thought, boy, I should have listened to my first instinct. I knew it wouldn't be good and it wasn't."

Sharon recalled a trip to Chicago when one of the tires blew and her husband's response. "He was really angry and upset — *not* because we were almost killed — but with *us*. He said to me, 'If you had been driving we would have been killed!' Then he blamed it on something my daughter, who was in the back seat, had done. My mother hated him; he was very mean to her. Of course, she's a lot like he is, so I kind of blew that off.

"In the time leading up to our marriage, he'd been positive about it in his own way — but then we're talking about somebody who can't express emotion. There were a couple of occasions when he'd displayed stern, highly critical behavior that I thought was almost over the edge. But we talked about our families — he had one child and I had three. We talked about taking vacations together. In fact, we had taken vacations together and things had gone well. They had been really fun.

"He told me a bit about his ex-wife. I do believe him when he says that she's an active drug addict, but much of the information he passed on about her to me was false. In fact, I think he absolutely lied. When I later found out the scope of his deception, I was incredulous. I had him on a pedestal. I couldn't believe how much he lied to me before we were married."

Sharon spoke candidly about her own addiction. "I was a Vicodin addict — I began using before I married him, but it got worse afterward (which was my choice). I had been using Vicodin for more than pain management. He found out because I had ordered some Vicodin online. I had my own mailbox, but a confirmation for an order showed up in his mailbox. He confronted me. I told him I only did it once — you know the old story — but then he told me he didn't believe me and I confessed. The night before, I had rolled over to turn the light off and said, 'God, please don't let me do this again,' and then the next day I was caught. That was it. I thought I was going to be out on the street that evening.

"When he caught me using, he was very unkind, partially because his ex-wife had an addiction. He told me to pack my bags and get out of the house. He was on the phone with attorneys immediately to see whether his license was compromised by my drug use. It was never a case of, 'Gee, I know you're sick, how can I help?' I was really physically extremely ill, because withdrawal from Vicodin is very unpleasant. He would take away all the charge cards, then give them back and take them away again. He'd accuse me of using when I really wasn't. Some of that I understand, because people have a hard time trusting, but he was so unkind — he was a verbal abuser.

"That summer, we went to San Francisco and took the kids; we traveled around some before going back into the city, where we spent the night before our plane left there. We checked into our hotel, and he said, 'I need to talk to you. How do you think this marriage is going?' I said, 'I think things are getting better.' He said, 'Well, I don't and I want a divorce.' There we were, on vacation with our kids, sitting in a hotel room! So I got a different room, took my kids there, and he told his daughter that I had a real self-esteem problem and that I had spent thousands of his dollars on my addiction — which was a lie. I later told his daughter the truth.

"The next day he met me at the airport, and he was contrite. When we got home, we went for a drive, and I told him this has got to stop. He said he'd never do it again. When I heard those words I should have *known* what I was in for, but I didn't. I asked him what he was going to tell his daughter, now that he'd defamed my character to her. He said he'd straighten it out."

They had been married three years at that point.

Sharon was never able to determine what sparked her husband's bizarre behavior, but speculates an addiction of his own had a lot to do with it.

"He was an addict, too — a sex addict — and the money he accused me of spending was going to that. He would carry over a thousand dollars cash at all times, telling me he needed it for Walmart, and so on. I was in such denial. He carried the checkbook in his briefcase all the time. I wasn't really healthy, and crossing boundaries I shouldn't, so I looked in there; I saw that he was taking out fifteen hundred to two thousand dollars a week. That isn't Walmart money! Then I saw where he had borrowed from our home improvement loan to pay his charge cards. He always presented himself as this great money manager, but I figured out that he wasn't managing the money at all.

"He'd already told me that he was going to Sex Addicts

Anonymous [SAA], but I knew he hadn't told me everything. I confronted him and asked him where the money was going. He told me he was having assignations with other women. That was it; I told him I was leaving."

It seems so simple in retrospect, but Sharon's path to that terminal moment was not an easy one. Her ex was a master manipulator whose control tactics had kept her off-balance for the duration of their relationship.

"At his suggestion, I stopped working after we got married, though I started again after the San Francisco incident," she recalled. "He would give me a set amount of money every week for the household expenses, and he controlled all the rest of the money. He didn't want to participate in decisions, though he'd make cracks about the decisions I made. I bought a vacuum; he told me months later that I had 'cleaned out his accounts' for that vacuum cleaner, and then never used it — which wasn't true."

Other forms of control emerged as well. "His daughter spent every other holiday with his mother. One year she was with her mother and he wasn't going to have Christmas with us because his daughter was gone. He was angry and wouldn't speak with us. He said I had no understanding or concern for his life and his problems, that I never supported him. Of course, he'd never told me any of the problems he was having, so how could I support him? Another time, he took my kids' CD players and threw them in the trash because he didn't think the kids were being kind and gracious enough.

"Another time, I was supposed to take my daughter and her friend to basketball camp. His daughter was with his ex, and she hadn't returned yet. He said, 'Angie isn't back and I don't know where she is.' I kind of snickered like, 'Yeah, I know,' because every time she left with her mother, we never got her back on time; it would take forever to get her back. But he was so angry at me for snickering that he wouldn't let me leave the house; he physically blocked my path so I couldn't leave the house to take my daughter and her friend to camp. He was a prick.

"He was into that 'violence of silence' thing with me, too, where he wouldn't speak to me, and *that* was very controlling. I broke my wrist once; he took me in for surgery and sat in a chair across from me and wouldn't speak to me while we were registering. He was working in the emergency room that night, and they wheeled me over to him. He called a neighbor to come and take me home. He went to work every day after that and left me alone, and never did anything to help me at home during my recovery.

"Once, I had a really bad migraine. Because of the Vicodin I had rebound headaches — but this one was severe; I was vomiting all day long. We went to the emergency room and he walked ten feet ahead of me; he left me to get sick in the middle of the sidewalk and just kept walking away from me. My self-esteem was so low, I just felt that I deserved it. He would do things when no one was around but me, and so I was left to figure it out for myself. But then my daughter told me he threw a laundry basket at her one day when they were alone. When I asked him about it, he told me he didn't want to talk about it — that what was done was done. He broke things of mine; we weren't allowed to touch his things. I think he poisoned my dog; the two times my dog was really ill he was alone with my husband, and I came home and found him very sick. I don't know the extent to which he would have gone."

On the job, Sharon's ex also exhibited control, but in a good way by being disciplined, diligent, thorough, and organized. At home, he was oblivious. "He could pass me in the hallway and not realize I was even there," she said. "He worked hard, and I think he thought it was beneath him to cook or clean. He didn't know what to do about it, and because of his addiction, he didn't want anyone to be in his home.

"He built this world of deceit. I'd see him begin to withdraw — for example, he'd sleep in a closet all of the time. He said it was because he worked nights and couldn't sleep otherwise. His closet was piled up on either side of where he slept with books and papers that dated back to the 1970s. Every once in a while, I would just gather up bags of trash and drag them out of there. This was a five-bedroom house. After we moved there, I noticed that his daughter would go to her room and close the door, and he would do the same. The doors were always closed.

"He is unkind in public, demeaning and demanding of people, and saying things solely to demoralize them. You get to the point where you can't answer his questions because he's just so inappropriate and he relied on that — at home as well. He would come up with these ridiculous statements and observations that simply stunned us.

"With people more powerful than him, he would only talk about medicine. We went to a fundraiser once, and no one would sit with us until there were absolutely no other seats available. An oncologist who finally sat next to us asked my husband, 'Can't we just talk about skiing or vacations or something other than medicine?' But my husband couldn't handle a social conversation."

In retrospect, Sharon still wonders why she stayed married to him as long as she did. The breaking point came when she began to fear for her children.

"With his addiction, I didn't want him around my daughter. She wouldn't back down [from a confrontation] and I was afraid she'd antagonize him, so my kids and I moved out and left his daughter to live with him. And they seem to be quite happy."

Even now, Sharon is confused as to why her ex-husband didn't just tell her he didn't want to get married in the first place. "Maybe he did try to tell me and I just didn't hear it. But he'd be so conciliatory whenever we had any disagreements. In the end, he did agree to marital counseling. But we are both very bright people, and we share so many interests — things you can't share with everyone else. For example, in the *New York Times*, we'd read the same obscure articles. I thought that we could work out our problems.

"But when he was already going to SAA, and then decided to break his 'sobriety,' I had to go. I knew that I would focus so much on his problem that I couldn't focus on mine, and that I would use his behavior as an excuse for my own, and I couldn't have that."

What advice would Sharon give others considering marriage to a doctor? "I would tell anyone to give it some serious thought. I'm sure there are some good doctor–wife relationships, but I haven't seen too many successful ones. I have a friend who was married to an OB/GYN; they had five children when he left her to marry a babysitter. He had two children with her, then started messing around with someone else, so she's now divorcing him.

"Some of the old family practice docs were well known to be carrying on with nurses in the hospital. There is a sense of entitlement, even down to the ones who seem the least likely. Doctors are hard to live with — demanding — and the public lets them get by with it.

"If I ever saw empathy from my husband, it was in response to someone who might come to the free clinic; someone who was totally downtrodden with horrid medical problems; someone who was so far beneath him that he could afford to have a moment of compassion for them. But he was terribly threatened by almost everyone else. People who know him are shocked that we were ever married. They wonder how he could live with anyone who simply knows how to lead a normal life and have a good time. And I can promise you that anyone who ever worked with him in the ER doesn't ever think about the fact that he gave the right diagnoses and treated patients correctly, but they *always* remember his cold demeanor."

"Margaret Anson" is a psychologist who has been in private practice for fifteen years. Her patients include older adolescents with eating disorders, women of all ages, and couples. Many have come from physicians' families, which gives her a particularly acute insight into what makes a lot of dysfunctional medical marriages tick — and survive.

"I see a lot of women patients who present with marital issues, many of them married to physicians. When they began to talk about their marriages, it became clear that their husbands might be having affairs. When I discussed that with them, the women would say, 'no, no, no'; but then, when the husbands came in, it was 'yes, yes, yes.' But most striking, these women were willing to stay in the marriage, tolerating disrespectful behavior because of financial concerns, status concerns, and concerns for their children."

Are many women more willing to remain in bad marriages when the spouse is a doctor or other high-profile professional than they would be if their husbands were, say, engineers or CPAs? Anson reply was an emphatic "yes."

"Often they are in awe of their husbands and their husbands' brilliance," she said. "Sometimes they *are* incredibly brilliant and accomplished, but the best of them have humility and honor their wives. I have a friend who is an incredibly successful physician, and he always cites his wife as the reason for that success.

"Some of these men, however, show some core personality traits that are associated with narcissistic behavior," she continued. "They do tremendous community work but treat their wives with only the minimum level of respect. The essence of narcissism is a failure to understand the effect of your actions on others. So these people can give tons of money to charity, do all of these wonderful things, and they don't really see a disconnect with how wonderful they are in those situations, and the way they treat their wives.

"They might say, 'Look at all I do for my wife! Look at the clothes she wears, the way we live, the trips we take, the house we live in, all of the wonderful things I make possible for her.' When I see them behave disrespectfully to their wives and confront them with it, they are totally oblivious. They feel entitled — the old 'princes of entitlement.' I can't say they have full-blown personality disorders, but they absolutely have these features. And why? Because they've been over-indulged by teachers, parents, society for so long that they live in a false world in terms of how they treat people."

As to the question of whether the medical training process can actually feed excessive ego, or whether many who are drawn to medicine have those tendencies in the first place, Anson has given that a great deal of thought.

"I've spent most of my adult life entertaining questions about that very issue — 'nature versus nurture.' Let me tell you an anecdote:

I had a patient who is a brilliant young woman and a physician. When she got to medical school, we were talking about a student of mine that she knew, and she said, 'Oh, he's great. He's not one of those typical arrogant, yuppie doctors who are in my medical school class.'

"But then I think about my husband and other physicians, and they absolutely must be clear, strong, and definite in their statements. Patients don't want to ask a doctor, 'Am I going to die?' and hear, 'Well, I don't know . . .' Doctors have to be very confident and assured to be effective. Some of the best doctors — those who are well known and achieve the most respect — are humble. While I do believe many people drawn to medicine are interested in helping others, it would be safe to say that in an earlier time it was true that people with narcissistic personalities were drawn to medicine."

In her clinical practice, Anson has noted that ego-driven, narcissistic behavior frequently is a source of conflict in marriages involving physicians or other high-powered professionals — one of the more common problems, in fact.

"Maybe that's changing now. Insurance companies are making it harder for doctors to earn so much money and limiting their autonomy. Team-oriented medicine, lower prestige, less autonomy — all are changing the dynamic of medicine as a career choice. I do think that younger women are more cognizant of the power thing in a marriage, and want to be married to someone who will honor them.

"You can't limit this idea to doctors alone, however," she emphasized. "Many psychologists or people who enter academia are incredibly narcissistic. The college professor who has numerous affairs with his students, for example, is exhibiting classic narcissistic behavior. The theory is that narcissistic men marry women with dependent personality disorders; these women are dependent to begin with so are drawn to the narcissistic man. For me, it's very hard just to limit the discussion solely to doctors.

"I find that wives of these driven professionals — like this subset of doctors who exhibit narcissistic traits — often feel very lonely, like second-class citizens in the family. Their marriages suffer from a lack of intimacy. The first few years are very exciting because they do things and go places, and there's status and prestige associated with being married to this person. But at some point they realize that they're not really talking to each other. He may consider his wife to be intellectually inferior, so he stops discussing things with her. Narcissists often think, 'Well, she just wouldn't understand.' "

Some highly driven professionals avoid their marriages through constant work, Anson said, citing as an example one client who had four graduate degrees, including one in law and two in medicine. "He worked constantly," she said, "but it was just avoidance. It was a turn-on to be so in demand and making so much money.

"The wives in these relationships feel lonely and have lives that lack intimacy. Often, as mothers, these women become overly involved with the children, and then the eating disorders piece comes into play.

"When wives are doing okay in these marriages, it's because they have really created their own life," Anson said. "Volunteer work, tennis, or whatever — because their husbands typically don't want them to work. Some of these women navigate their world through incredible participation in volunteer activities. I was in Junior League in a former life, and that organization had a number of women who had created a busy life for themselves. But for me, the sadness of their situation was they didn't have a true partner. I always think relationships depend first on a true partnership.

"So many of these women create a life molded around their husbands instead of creating a life that is about their own passions and dreams. When they come to me I ask, 'What are you passionate about? What do you care about?' In the case of one couple, in which the husband was having an affair and the wife was in denial about it, she couldn't think of anything that was *her* passion. Everything connected to him. That marriage ended eventually, which wasn't surprising."

What about cases in which the *woman's* narcissism sparks problems in a marriage? "Well, oddly enough," Anson said, "the women I have counseled — who as a society we would say are high-powered professionals — are all divorced. If you look at divorce, and particularly at John Gottman's work with couples [Gottman is a psychologist whose studies have focused on marital stability and relationship analysis], you find that most women married to a narcissist will put up with that for a very long time. If the narcissistic husband doesn't know his wife's dreams or isn't interested in her opinion, the couple can stay married for a long time, then perhaps divorce later on.

"Where the woman is the more aggressive and power-centered, however, those couples get divorced early on."

Anson spoke frankly of the challenges facing any marriage involving a narcissistic partner. "Awareness is critical. When you get into a relationship, and you see the red flags of narcissism — egotism, lack of empathy, and so on — you must talk about it. But you can't cure true NPD. Those men or women can, through therapy or through losing a relationship, become aware of what they do. I've had men say, 'I know I'm a narcissist.' Some women are strong enough to call their husbands on this behavior, too. If you love a person, you might be able to survive that. But the thing with personality disorders in general is that you're seeking awareness and mindfulness, not a 'cure.' For narcissistic doctors, they need to realize that they do a lot for society, but they need to bring some of that good treatment home.

"All that said," Anson added, "if you're dealing with someone who truly is narcissistic with NPD, I doubt that the marriage can be saved. The compromise and sacrifice is just too great, unless that other partner is willing to have a roommate rather than a spouse, and do their own thing with their life. Often the first step in healing a couple is to ask them to stop looking at each other and start looking back at themselves as individuals, to discover what kinds of changes they need to make.

"So often for women, that involves taking a job, getting involved in volunteer work, returning to a long-neglected passion for painting, and so on. Then, the husband with narcissistic traits sees that his wife is no longer blaming him, no longer living through him — she's taking care of herself. And at that point, the husband can say, 'Maybe I need to start taking care of myself and stop looking at her for a solution.'

"One woman I met with is married to a narcissist, and I had to tell her straightforwardly, 'This man is not going to change. You have to look at this marriage and decide, is this enough for a lifetime? Can you continue to share a life with someone who behaves this way?' Ultimately, that's the decision spouses of truly narcissistic people have to make."

. . . AND AT WORK

If narcissistic Doctor Gods are tough to be married to and live with, what's it like to work with them?

I clearly recall a time when doctors were the undisputed lords of their realm. Those days are gone. As mentioned earlier in this book, a number of factors — including insurance oversight and managed-care operations, changes in employment status, and a shift toward team medicine — combined to topple them from their thrones.

Insurance oversight and its influence must rank first among the factors reducing physician autonomy in the workplace. Many treatments now must be pre-approved, requiring incredible administrative accountability and clearances. A number of physicians have opted out of the insurance system entirely, strictly to avoid the time, expense, and frustration of submitting claims for payment. Their patients are left to pay for treatment themselves, then submit their own claims and deal with the hassles that follow. In either event, the system has interfered with a doctor's unfettered ability to call the shots in his or her practice.

Another factor that has taken away some of the control that doctors used to enjoy is their state of employment. Throughout the twentieth century most doctors were self-employed. By 2001, however, over a third of all physicians were employees of hospitals, clinics, and managed-care providers. In any field, being an employee, rather than a one-person shop, has some benefits, but it also means sacrificing some independence. Clinic and hospital policies influence everything from the amount of time doctors can spend with patients to the types of treatments they can prescribe, which therefore gives doctors less control over their practices. (Of course, even those doctors who remain their own boss are under the whip of price and time controls, as they must earn enough to pay the costs of running their businesses.)

Team medicine is the norm in many medical facilities today, and doctors are called upon to function within that capacity. Nurses and other medical staff now perform many of the procedures that used to be handled exclusively by doctors, thus increasing physicians' reliance on their support staff more than ever — and that requires maintaining good working relationships.

Nor is it as common for administrators to turn a blind eye to outbursts of abusive physician behavior, such as screaming at medical assistants or throwing charts at nurses (although, according to some, those behaviors haven't disappeared entirely). These hospitals and clinics require that doctors work cooperatively with other staff members; those who don't often find themselves reprimanded or brought before review committees.

Mention "Doctor God" to practicing physicians and medical educators, and you'll likely hear that he's quickly disappearing from the scene, thanks to new training approaches, changing attitudes toward medicine, and shifting demographics (in other words, more women and minorities) within the medical profession. Nevertheless, when most patients and nurses speak about the doctors they work with, it becomes apparent that, although dwindling in numbers, Doctor Gods continue to stalk the halls of clinics and hospitals across the country.

In fact, many medical facilities have been forced to come to grips with the issue of doctors behaving badly — a problem that's come to be known as "disruptive physician behavior." As the hierarchy within the field of medicine shifts, as our nation's nursing shortage deepens, and as workers in every field demand more protection from the stresses of a hostile work environment, medical administrators find themselves both unable and unwilling to put up with abusiveness in the workplace. With some areas predicting that one in four nursing slots will go unfilled by the year 2020, we all desperately want the field to remain attractive to those who feel called to service. Getting abusive doctors to clean up their acts is an important step toward that goal.

DOCTOR–NURSE RELATIONSHIPS

Among the most critical things impacting patient care today is the doctor–nurse relationship. Like the field of medicine itself, that relationship has undergone some change over the past hundred years, but that change has been less dramatic than you might suppose. In the early twentieth century, nurses were considered to be little more than medicine's handmaidens whose workplace status was driven by issues of both gender and class; the vast majority of doctors were affluent males, and an even larger majority of nurses were women from middle- or working-class families. Nurses were expected to treat each doctor with absolute deference, rising when he entered a room, using his full title when addressing him, and never forgetting that she was simply a mechanism for carrying out his orders. As J. McGregor-Robinson, MD, wrote in 1902 about the role of the trained nurse in health care delivery, "...she occupies no independent position in the treatment of the sick person."

Throughout much of the twentieth century, nurses were expected to refrain from expressing medical opinions to patients. In 1967, psychiatrist Leonard Stein referred to the "doctor–nurse game" as an unspoken arrangement by which nurses expressed observations or made suggestions to doctors in passive ways that enabled the doctors to feel they had ownership over the ideas. Historically, for example, nurses learned to describe their observations of patients' conditions to doctors in nonclinical terms so as not to appear to be assuming medical authority or knowledge. According to Suzanne Gordon, in her acclaimed book *Nursing Against the Odds: How Health Care Cost Cutting, Media Stereotypes, and Medical Hubris Undermine Nurses and Patient Care*, the practice of using the "nursing diagnoses" — which is still taught in many nursing schools — is little more than a standardization of the linguistic sidestepping nurses adopted historically to help avoid treading on doctors' toes.

In 1990, Stein released a follow-up report on his earlier study. In "The Doctor–Nurse Game Revisited," Stein and his colleagues reported that nurses were no longer willing to be silent servants in patient health care. "New" nurses were bold and vocal, Stein stated, and more than willing to voice their opinions or challenge a doctor's decisions. To many in health care, these findings signaled a movement toward strengthening the role of teamwork in patient care, and as such, good news for doctors, nurses, and patients alike.

Just twelve years later, however, when Alan Rosenstein, medical director of a regional division of VHA, Inc. (a national network of community-owned hospitals and heath-care systems) did his own original research into the state of doctor–nurse relationships in that system, he didn't find much evidence of good news. Rosenstein's survey revealed that over 92 percent of all respondents had witnessed disruptive physician behavior, which they cited as physicians yelling or raising their voices, being disrespectful or condescending, berating colleagues and patients, and using abusive language. While the survey's participants reported that this behavior occurred in no more than 3 percent of the medical staff, they still considered it a real problem. On a scale of 1 to 10, nurses and administrators rated the severity of the problem of disruptive physician behavior at 7.13 and 7.85 respectively. Doctors rated it at less than 6.

The three groups also had differing views on the triggers for disruptive behavior. Nurses said that they most frequently encountered outbursts when they placed a call to a physician; asked for clarification of the physician's orders; when the physician felt that his or her orders weren't being carried out as quickly as they should be; or after a sudden change in a patient's status. Doctors reported that such behavior occurred when orders weren't carried out correctly, when they received a call at an inconvenient time, or when nurses hadn't checked existing information before calling. Hospital executives agreed that disruptive behavior was often triggered by orders not being carried out to the physician's satisfaction, but added that the behavior also occurred as a result of "physicians not getting their way or not having their preferences met."

Although they may have different understandings of the severity of the problem, physicians, nurses, and administrators agree that poor communications and hostile working relationships have an impact on the attitudes of staff members throughout the hospital. By contributing to on-the-job dissatisfaction and burnout among qualified nursing and other medical staff, that impact extends to patient safety and outcomes.

Throughout the country, we're suffering from a shortage of well-trained, well qualified nurses — the nurses who are least likely to endure the rantings and temper tantrums of a Doctor God. According to a report released by the American Association of Colleges of Nursing, as many as 55 percent of surveyed nurses say they plan to retire between 2011 and 2020. In Rosenstein's survey, 30 percent of respondents said that they knew of nurses leaving their hospitals as a result of disruptive behavior.

Currently, new enrollees in nursing programs are declining, as are the number of qualified nursing instructors. As a result, the average age of RNs in America is increasing, right along with the number of our nation's elderly population. Most of us have grown tired of hearing about the needs of the aging baby-boomer generation, but good nursing care is going to top the list. According to the Joint Commission on Accreditation of Healthcare Organizations (JCAHO), by 2020 our nation will have 400,000 fewer nurses than will be needed to care for our population. A shortage of nurses results in compromised patient care. The JCAHO examined over sixteen hundred reports of "sentinel events" — unanticipated events that resulted in hospital patient deaths and injuries — and found that staffing levels were directly tied to nearly a quarter of all cases.

High turnover rates in nursing also add greatly to the cost of health care and drive down the profitability of the institutions that provide it. Some sources estimate that organizations spend the equivalent of an average annual nursing salary to replace one nurse. For a hospital with a staff of 600 nurses, those replacement costs can amount to over $5.5 million dollars *per year*.

These side effects of a poor working environment for nurses — compromised patient care, reduced access to health care, and a health care system that grows more expensive even as it becomes less effective — give us all a stake in the health of the typical doctor–nurse relationship.

In its report, the JCAHO made three recommendations for addressing the nursing shortage; the first among these was to retain trained nursing staff by fostering a workplace that is respectful of nursing and by adopting "zero tolerance policies for abusive behaviors by health care practitioners." In the United States, England, Canada, India, Norway — even Trinidad and Tobago — reports of physician abuse continue to spark debate about the need for new programs to combat such behavior.

The evidence seems clear that peer review isn't always effective in controlling doctor behavior. As a result, institutions have had to find their own methods for regulating physician behavior. The official descriptions of these programs typically emphasize their role in improving "patient safety" or "physician–nurse collaboration," but most are built around a central set of policies for tracking and controlling abusive physician behavior.

No matter how well we construct systems for controlling physician behavior, no system will work if administrators refuse to enforce its guidelines. In Alan Rosenstein's 1990 survey, nearly two-thirds of all respondents confirmed that code-of-conduct policies were in place at their hospital, yet fewer than half of the respondents thought those policies were effective. While a majority of respondents agreed they could file reports of disruptive behavior without fear of punishment, nearly half of them admitted that there were barriers to reporting. In this group, nurses reported that the barriers included intimidation, fear of retaliation, and/or damage to future relationships. Some feared legal consequences.

These fears are understandable, even today. Some of the nurses we spoke with said that even though their hospitals did have policies governing disruptive behavior, they didn't believe those policies could really protect them from physicians who were big money-makers for the hospital. Popular surgeons generate incredible revenues for a hospital, and nurses may rightly believe that an arrogant, even abusive, surgeon will be protected from administrative reprimands by his or her profitability.

Disruptive physician behavior doesn't begin in the workplace, any more than do the attitudes that feed such behavior. Doctors in training often learn the politics of workplace harassment during their internships. According to one study, by the time they entered their senior year of clinical rotations, nearly three out of every four U.S. medical students surveyed reported that they had been harassed or belittled by residents. Dr. Erica Frank, one of the study's authors and vice chairwoman of Atlanta's Emory University School of Medicine, said: "We give a lot of lip service to teaching professionalism [and] to reducing the prevalence of disruptive physicians . . ." but then went on to stress that until we specifically train doctors *not* to exhibit this kind of behavior, we won't make much progress in changing the culture of medicine that supports it.

As noted earlier, Indiana University School of Medicine's competency-based curriculum and its components stress professionalism in dealing with patients, nurses, and other staff. The University of Kentucky takes another educational approach toward this goal with its Registered Nurse–Resident Physician Preceptorship Program. In this program, new residents are paired with registered nurses in eight-hour shifts, giving residents an opportunity to fully appreciate nurses' functions and the contributions they make in the health-care process. By creating more common ground and shared understanding between doctors and nurses, these and other programs like them strive to improve the doctor–nurse collaboration.

DOCTOR DICTATORS

We met Sharon earlier, a woman who had a brief and unhappy marriage to an emergency room physician. Because she also worked thirty years as a registered nurse in hospital settings, she has had a lifetime of professional experience with doctors of all types. As an emergency room nurse, Sharon works in what many describe as a hotbed for disruptive physician behavior. She shared a glimpse of a typical day in a community hospital ER.

"Generally, the nursing staff comes to work and does their thing; the physician is already there, depending on the shift. The doc sees patients and gives orders and we implement them. We discharge the patients when the doctor doesn't want to go back in and deal with them. Often, when there's a code, the nursing staff runs that and the docs will just come in and make sure that everything is okay, concentrating their time on other things. When things get hectic, it gets more hectic for the physician than the nursing staff because people are waiting to see the doc all the time. Sometimes the docs get real short-tempered and snap."

Sharon had described her husband as controlling, dismissive, and autocratic — a true Doctor God — but he wasn't the only doctor Sharon encountered who shared these personality traits. "I've run into several like him," she told us. "I had a doctor throw a chart at me once. When later complaining about me to my boss, he said that if I were standing there with them at that moment, he would hit me. I've seen less of that behavior in the professional setting than I used to, though. I've seen it changing — not in the old docs, but in the new ones. I see them misbehave, but it's not routine; at least it's not as obvious. The hospitals have measures in place to stop that kind of mistreatment now. The nurses report abusive behavior and a board investigates it. We didn't used to have that kind of support — but if it came down to 'him or me,' they would believe the doctor."

Sharon believes a number of factors are at work to reduce abusive behavior in the medical workplace. "There's been a change in the way hospitals oversee doctors. Many doctors are employees of the hospital and under the same scrutiny as any other employee. The loss of independence is changing things, too. They're not the king of the hill anymore. And there are more female doctors. I don't see this behavior as often among female physicians. I've seen it in older female physicians, but not as much in the younger ones. Do I think it still exists? Absolutely. When push comes to shove, doctors will pull rank.

"We have an ER physician who's female. She was one of the first female ER physicians in the country and she's a tough nut to crack. When she didn't want to do something, she wouldn't do it. We were supposed to do employee health physicals, and she didn't want to do them. When I went to work at the hospital, I sat there for *three hours* waiting for her to do my physical, and she finally told me she wasn't going to do it. I went to the administration and told them that she was refusing to give me a physical — I wasn't going to argue with her. And she'd make patients wait forever. The patients would be waiting and she'd be back there brushing her teeth."

While women are making inroads into the medical workplace, Sharon still sees gender inequities in patients' treatment.

"Pain management has become a very difficult process in the ER right now. We have a lot of people with drug-seeking behavior, and we also have some with a very legitimate need for drugs. Distinguishing between them can be difficult. My ex-husband is very unsympathetic with pain, especially in women. And there's another ER doc that's just like that. Men can come in and get the pain medicine they need, but not the women. Men in particular like to think that women are just emotional and exaggerating their pain. That attitude is pervasive in our society and among many male doctors."

Sharon understands the dilemma doctors face when trying to evaluate patients' need for pain relief. "You also see many women come in who have a lot of other dynamics going on, and you can't really tell whether their pain is physical or psychological. It's interesting, however, that the doctors tend to question pain more for women rather than men."

Distressed-physician behavior has a real impact on nurses —

and patient care. "I've never had too much trouble, because I won't let it happen," Sharon told us. "But they'll harass anyone who is the least bit timid. And patient care gets compromised. If patients are not doing well or unsure [about the patient's condition], timid nurses won't call the doctor, especially not in the middle of the night. I say, 'That's what they're being paid for.' So I call them, and if they hang up on me I call them back. Sometimes they'll say, 'What do you want me to do?' And I'll say, 'I want you to come here and see if this patient is alright; I want you to come and tell me whether what I'm seeing is a problem or not. You're his doctor!'"

This scenario sets up a real internal conflict for nurses, who hesitate to tell a patient that he or she is getting substandard care from a physician, but at the same time, can't just sit back and watch the problems unfold. Sharon has her own method for dealing with this situation. "I will tell patients that we have contacted their doctor and their doctor has not responded, and that as a patient, it's their right to call him themselves. The doctors hate it when their patients call them from the hospital, and/or seek another caregiver. But these days, we have a house physician who will take care of things when the regular doc is unavailable."

Sharon believes that the old ego-driven Doctor God behavior is diminishing but still factors in most medical workplaces. She also understands its roots. "I think they [doctors] have to have a little of that in order to survive. They have to believe in themselves. But I believe doctors do think that they're a step above everyone else. And you know the public gives them that. I had a friend once say to me, 'But look at it, they have lives in their hands, of course they're going to feel like God.' And I said, 'Excuse me, but they don't have people's lives in their hands that often if they're doing the right thing. And let's face it, I'm the one doing CPR in the emergency room, not the doctors. If lives are in anyone's hands, they're in mine.' But medicine is not an exact science, and I do think that doctors have to believe that they make better decisions. You can't second-guess yourself or take your problems home with you."

The ER could be considered the most stressful place in a

hospital at times, but probably the most stressful and demanding collaborations exist in the operating rooms between surgeons and operating room nurses. "Madeline," an experienced OR nurse at a mid-sized hospital in the Midwest, concurs. At the age of thirty-nine, Madeline went back to school and got her nursing degree. After graduation, Madeline took a job as a student nurse in the hospital where she continues to work today.

Advanced technology is what first attracted Madeline to working in the OR. "I had been on the table on many occasions, and I knew it made a difference if someone was there to hold your hand and reassure you as you went under anesthesia," she said. "There are studies showing that the more relaxed you are when you are going under anesthesia, the more easily you'll come out of it. If I can make someone smile when they're in trouble, I feel like I've done my job for the day. When people talk about *nursing*, they're talking about helping and reassuring people in their worst, most fearful times."

Madeline works the evening shift. Her typical workday in the OR begins at 3 P.M., when she changes into her scrubs and checks the assignment schedule to see where she'll be working. Then the fun begins.

"Taking care of cases depends on what duty you have — scrubbing in and helping surgeons, either by passing instruments or assisting with actual surgery," she explained. "Or we take care of the room, fill out paperwork, and so on, which is called circulating. As a circulator, I will go over and get the patient from the holding area. I have six or seven forms I have to fill out. I go in and talk to the patient, ask some simple questions — when was the last time you ate, what consents have you signed, and so on. I assess skin color, temperature, IV sites, nausea. Then, I take the patient into the room and help the anesthesiologists intubate by watching monitors while he's doing things or when he leaves the room. The minute the anesthesiologist leaves, I'm responsible for the monitors. The patients feel a lot of reliance on us. I always introduce patients to all of the staff, but I'm the one who talks to the patient. I even try to kid them if it's appropriate. You have to read people."

Although she received little student training as an OR nurse, Madeline quickly learned the politics of her profession once she began work. "As a student, I spent just one day in the OR. The six months of orientation, *that's* where I learned what it was really like. I remember, I went into a room to observe. And the surgeon who was in there . . . I was so totally blown away by the way he was treating the people in the room. He talked down; he was degrading. In our post-conference after that day, I said, 'I am appalled at the way he talked and treated people, and the way he talked about his patients.' But everyone else seemed to think nothing unusual had happened. I guess you get used to it after a while.

"Of course, it depends on what surgeon you're working with. Some are notoriously temperamental — real Doctor God types. I would say you have maybe half of them who can be really tyrannical; the other half are thoughtful and tell you they appreciate your work. You see disruptive behavior more often in older rather than younger surgeons. When they [the younger surgeons] start, it's like, 'Wow, they're so nice!' Then the older surgeons mentor them and you see the transformation take place. We have hardly any female surgeons — three women out of thirty-five total surgeons. I work with one female surgeon who was a nurse for eleven years, then went to school to become a doctor. She's wonderful. She has an empathy and understanding for what it's like to work with doctors.

"But with many, you see your assignment and just say, 'Oh my God, I don't want to work with him.' A lot of nurses just don't want to be in the room with them. You get in there and just hope nothing malfunctions — that the scissors are sharp, for example — because we'll take the heat for that even though we aren't responsible. I was in one room where the surgeon took a laparoscopic instrument, bent it in half, and threw it across the room.

"They cuss, too. I was really surprised at the language they use. Sometimes it's directed toward us, other times toward the situation. I had a surgeon call me a 'stupid fuck' once. In this case, it was totally out of character for this surgeon. I think his frustration came from somewhere else, and it was just a fluke. I didn't report it, but someone else in the room did. Then my supervisor came to me and said I needed to write a report on it. I said I wasn't really willing to do that because it was a lapse for him, not a way of behavior."

Madeline also acknowledged that not much happens as a result of these write-ups.

"It goes on their record, but if they're making money for your hospital, bottom line rules. For example, we have a bariatric surgeon who . . . well, I don't like to be in his room — ever. He gets on a tear and you have to walk on eggshells around him. He threw a nurse out of the room the other day. He doesn't want fat nurses in his room, either, and he makes it known. He's been talked to by administration and he'll be on his best behavior for a few weeks, then it spirals back out of control. They won't do more than talk to him. He's an excellent surgeon and makes so much money for the hospital that they don't come down too hard. If you tell a PCC [Patient Care Coordinator, the direct supervisor of nurses in Madeline's hospital] that a doctor was rude to you, the PCC will defend the doctor by saying he was stressed out or whatever. They want to keep the doctors happy."

Madeline understands that good surgeons require a certain level of confidence, but she sees a big difference in self-confident action and egotistical bullying.

"I think you have to have a certain type of personality to be a surgeon; you have to think that you're the best there is, not just an 'okay' surgeon. But then you have surgeons who think they're the greatest, and I wouldn't take my dog to them, and some are like Jekyll and Hyde. As their patients, people will say, 'Oh, he's such a wonderful man — I have such complete confidence in him.' And I think, *Are you kidding?* because when those patients are asleep on the operating table, you hear the doctor speaking very unkindly about them. That whole thing makes me wonder. When you have a bariatric surgeon who doesn't like fat people, it's kind of an odd occupational choice, isn't it?"

When recklessly egotistical behavior enters the operating room, disasters can unfold. Madeline has witnessed more than her share of such incidents.

"One of the worst Doctor God stories I know is of a man who came into the emergency room who had been bitten twice by a brown recluse spider. He waited and didn't come in to the ER until it was bad. Everyone who gets bitten by a brown recluse has a reaction, but some have an allergic reaction. This man's flesh was dying; overnight it started creeping, and he had flesh-eating bacteria. He came in on a Thursday morning, and by that evening, he had necrotizing fasciitis [serious infection of the deeper layers of the skin and subcutaneous tissue].

"I had been up in the intensive care unit helping another doctor, and I heard that we had a guy coming to surgery who was bad. I walked by his room and glanced in and saw the man, whose body was turning a purplish color. I knew he wasn't going to make it; he was too ravaged. It was a lost cause before they ever got him in there."

When Madeline later entered the operating room to assist in this patient's surgery, what she saw horrified her. "They had amputated one leg and taken out most of his belly and chest," she remembers. "They had split his arms from the shoulder to the wrist and were getting ready to amputate the other leg — they were still working on him! He was losing unbelievable amounts of blood. I tried to help straighten out the room, because it was crazy. I couldn't believe they had even started it. There was not going to be anything left of this man. He would never have survived surgery.

Madeline shuddered at the recollection, then continued.

"But we had a vascular surgeon who was one of these 'God' types, and it seemed like it was some kind of experiment for him: 'I can try this, I can try that.' I think he just wanted the experience. Of course, the general surgeon was taking out the stomach muscles and so on; everything was open, and he was just trying to keep up. The vascular surgeon kept saying, 'We can do this.' At the end, he finally realized that all he had was a heap of body parts and flesh, and he couldn't save the man. That surgery alone probably cost $115,000. We had a blood shortage, and we were throwing blood at someone who would never live — and the surgeon didn't care. It wasn't like he was trying to help this man and his family. It was like, '*I'M going to SAVE this man!*' I see that image as clearly as if it were today.

"That was where I saw Doctor God. That vascular surgeon was like that in many cases. For any vascular problem, surgery was the first choice. We used to joke that he cruised the emergency room to find someone to operate on. If someone came in with bad pulses in their feet, he'd be doing a bypass graft immediately. The next time you'd see him, they'd be amputating the patient's feet. It's a big power rush to do surgery, and these docs start to think they're the power.

"I talked to him about it once, kind of joking: 'Do you just hang out in the ER waiting for something to come along you can do surgery on?' He sort of grinned at me and said, 'Well, more and more people are having vascular disease — especially in the Midwest. They don't take care of themselves or eat right.' He said it was the patients' fault that he had to do this — like he had to come in and save all of these stupid people from themselves."

Thankfully, Madeline noted, the Doctor Gods are balanced by a host of truly terrific ones.

"We have one doctor, a nephrologist. We take out kidneys and so on, and he always lets me know that he is glad I'm in the room. He'll say, 'Man, it's good to see you in here.' He can be temperamental without being cruel. He rarely, if ever, loses his temper — and that's a good thing. You work with him and do your job and he appreciates it. When the case is done he'll come up and thank you and tell you that you did a good job. That just makes my day — to have someone tell me I'm doing a good job. We have an eye surgeon who mainly does cataract surgery and he always comes up to people and gives them a one-armed hug and thanks them for doing a good job, tells us we make *his* job easier."

Madeline's profession is demanding, but she is proud of it. "My niece told me she wanted to be a nurse, or maybe a surgical tech. I asked her why. 'If it's money, there are easier ways to earn it,' I told her, 'but if you want to help people, then yeah, go into it.' No matter what else happens at work, I can still have a good one-on-one with my patients and know that I made a difference. I do the extras. I go back and check on my patients when they're awake, and tell them they did well, and so on. I'll even go in the waiting room, when the case is over and I know the spouse has been really distraught. I assure them that everything went well, give them a hug, and tell them it will be okay.

"But that's just the way I do things. I consider I have my own nursing practice and nobody can take that away from me. That's why I stay in it. I see people at their very worst, and I tell them, 'You are my patient from now on.' I tell them to hold my hand, I offer to pray with them if they want. I've had people say, 'You're my angel; I couldn't have gone through this without you.' I absolutely love my work."

Nevertheless, Madeline is painfully aware of the politics that continue to govern the surgical workplace.

"It's the corporate game, with an emphasis on the bottom line and the idea that minimum care is okay because you just have to get the basics done — just what you can get charted. You can't chart that you sat with a patient and held their hand while they died, or talked with the family. And that's what nursing is — not charting.

"I love my work," she reiterated, "and I would like to stay with the company, but it's changed a lot since I've been there. A private company owns the hospital — we have several hospitals in the area. But we've had a lot of problems. We have an interim manager right now; they came in and made a lot of changes, got rid of a lot of people that they now realize we need. So now we're restaffing, and it takes six months to train in new people. It's a strange situation."

She paused and thought for a moment. "The day before yesterday," she said, "I walked into work and there was a magazine article posted on the bulletin board about medical bullying, and it specifically addressed behavior in the operating room. I read the first page, and it talked about all these stories; I didn't have time to finish the article, because I had to get back to work. The next day, I went in and it was gone. Someone took it off the bulletin board. I thought that was as interesting as the article. Obviously, someone thought that article shouldn't be posted for us to read."

DOCTORS BEGIN TO LEARN
THERE'S NO "I" IN "TEAM"

For many physicians, becoming effective members of a health-care team requires a significant learning curve. Franklin McKinzie counsels those who work in medicine and helps coach doctors to achieve that goal.

McKinzie is well qualified for such a position. He holds a doctorate in ministerial counseling and worked for fifteen years at a large metropolitan hospital as a pastoral counselor in the mental health center. He also has worked in an independent center counseling doctors faced with treating patients who are beyond traditional medical or surgical care.

"Although many doctors see themselves as being 'the boss,'" McKinzie noted, "some of them are ill-equipped to be effective leaders. Their approach is that, when they hear a problem, they try to fix it. A true team member knows when to step up and when to step back. Leadership involves listening to learn and asking to empower. Many doctors have trouble with that. They tend either to be micromanagers or to avoid management altogether and just let things happen. Medical school doesn't offer much training in leadership or management, so they have to just learn that on their own.

McKinzie thinks few doctors truly fit the Doctor God stereotype. "I've seen very dictatorial doctors, but they're in the minority. They create the most fuss, though, because the hospitals and CEOs have to deal with them, and they're difficult to deal with. Maybe one in ten doctors falls into that Doctor God type, but that one will cause all the problems, trying to dominate everyone else. It takes only one in ten to cause havoc in the workplace — or to ruin a marriage, for that matter."

Citing a book called *Trust and Betrayal in the Workplace*,

McKinzie pointed out three things people trust: Clear expectations, clear communication, and competence.

"If you don't provide those things," he said, "you have a broken trust. People who have the Doctor God syndrome are so locked into what they think is competent and how they should communicate that they don't tend to build trust with others because they fail to honor the expectations, communications, and competence of others. If you have the Doctor God syndrome, you're not going to listen to anyone else. You're going to just cut it out to fix it. Doctor Gods expect people to inherently trust them, but they won't build trust, so people have to buckle under to that doctor's will."

McKinzie has faced a number of challenges in helping physicians learn to be part of a functional team, the first of which "is getting them to recognize that they need to be helped, rather than be the helpers. I've had success working with them through a coaching model, which has more acceptance with these guys than does a traditional counselor."

To some doctors, McKinzie believes, having to meet with consultants implies that they've really become dysfunctional; but many now will hire an executive coach to help them learn how to develop an effective management style.

"Of course," he said, "the people who really need help — many of these doctors who have flashes of anger or a fight-or-flight response when things don't go their way — those guys don't hire me. The hospital CEOs hire me.

"One doctor I trained to be a coach liked the idea when we were training, but it was really tough for him to be calm when things went against what he wanted or thought should be done. Usually the issues had to do with money, and that can be perceived as a threat. If someone threatens these doctors' income, authority, or chosen processes, they become difficult to work with. They perceive a threat and they get into the anger zone. When that happens, I ask them to evaluate whether or not they've really been threatened. If it isn't a true threat they're facing, I teach them what to do rather than speaking to counter the problem: Listen to learn about the situation, rather than trying to 'hear and fix' or 'tell and solve.' These doctors are hearing you, but in their mind they're planning their rebuttal. Doctors like this aren't functional. They don't listen well. If there's a threat, they will simply get angry or dictatorial and scare people away. And that's when they appear to be Doctor God."

McKinzie has found a growing interest among doctors in learning coaching and leadership skills, simply because doctors know they have to be different from what they've been before.

"I think the people who go to medical school are very intelligent people who want to make a difference," McKinzie suggests. "The majority of doctors I know have a great deal of compassion, but I think that something happens in the process that makes them feel that they have to do this kind of [autocratic] thing. Anyone who works in a hospital has to have a way to deal with the traumatic experience of people in suffering and in pain and dying. And I don't want to share a decision with a brain surgeon; I don't want him to have a coaching role. I just want him to know what to do and do it. But then there are times where doctors have to be a coach — like when they work with people on adopting a better diet. If the doctor doesn't switch to the coach routine to help you with that, he won't succeed.

"There are three important questions we all must deal with," he concluded, "and those are: Who am I? Where am I going? Who am I going with? If you get those questions in the wrong order, you can't have a successful life. Doctor God is someone who says, 'Here's where we're going, and here's what we're going to do.' People who think that way forget who they are. They get the questions in the wrong order. Doctors who get it right have a synergy with their patients and their families and they work together."

Although many medical workplaces now have employee counseling programs in place to help nurses deal with abusive doctors and other problems, many nurses also turn to private therapists for help. Robin

Rossman is one such counselor. A nurse with an advanced practice degree in community mental health nursing, Rossman has worked for fifteen years in nurse training, consultation, and private practice. As a therapist and employee assistance counselor, she helps nurses deal with work–life problems and heal from traumas associated with their stressful career.

"I've counseled with a number of nurses who are trying to manage their career around doctors who display disruptive or negative behavior," she noted. "These nurses report a continuum of problems — beginning with a lack of empathy and a feeling that nurses or other health care professionals in a hospital setting are subservient. Doctors aren't keyed into an awareness that support personnel are essential. For years we've talked about being a team, but we've also seen that certain physicians are oblivious to the concept of teamwork including them. They view themselves as being 'the boss,' not a team member, although that attitude is changing quickly.

"On the continuum of disruptive behavior, that's one end. The other can be up to and including abusive behavior or an MD who truly is narcissistic. I've talked to a number of nurses who have described sexually inappropriate and demeaning behavior — doctors calling nurses idiots and other names. And I distinguish here between the everyday working relationship versus a true crisis. If you have someone who is dying, communication is secondary to the action that you're taking. People are forgiven for four-letter words and name-calling in a crisis.

"In the past, that kind of narcissistic behavior was role modeled. In students, for example, I can remember going through nursing training and watching the rounds and the physician with his entourage of students, residents, and interns pass through the hall. It was like the Red Sea parting. Certain physician educators would bully students and embarrass them, and I think they thought that was just the way you learned. They would put students on the spot either in front of the patient or in the hall in front of their peers. I think it was handed down as a tradition. But things are gradually changing, and we're already beginning to see more communication and honesty between doctors and patients, and maybe even a lessening in medical errors."

So how do most nurses deal with bullying behavior in doctors when they encounter it? "Many ignore it," Rossman said. "They rationalize it by saying, 'Well, that's just how he is, he's an asshole, or this thing or that thing.' Depending on the individuals and what kind of coping skills they have, nurses can be assertive. Some — especially those older, more educated, and more experienced — can confront bullying doctors. But it has a lot to do with the nurse's self-esteem. I'd like to think we have a lot of nurses who will sit down with the doctor and tell him that they won't accept abusive behavior. For the most part, however, they tolerate, ignore, and bear it.

"Nurses do an outstanding job of 'taking it' and not transferring their problems to their work. They get sick, get headaches, gain weight, become addicted, go home and kick the cat — they don't always deal with it in healthy ways. They'll even defend the doctor to the patient because they know the patient has to trust and believe in the doctor. Nurses will say to patients, 'You have the best doctor, don't worry.' In a way, it's like being the wife in an abusive marriage; you've got your kids, and even if your husband is abusive, you know that your kids need to believe in and obey their father, so you defend him to the kids."

Rossman has seen some positive changes in this pattern, however. "Historically, nurses did take a professional risk [if they reported a doctor for abusive behavior]. In the last several years this has changed because nurses are beginning to litigate against bullying doctors in the hospital. Doctors bring in the money, so hospitals walked the line, not wanting to alienate them. But things are shifting today *because* of the bottom line. Today, health-care employees have a different understanding of violence in the workplace. In the past, those workers considered that bullying was simply the terrain of health care; even if it created somatic physical ailments or even if they developed post-traumatic stress disorder (PTSD), that was the way it was. Now, employees are beginning to shift their assumptions about how much of this behavior you need to tolerate."

She also cites several changes in the typical physician's personality and behavior today. "Doctors are a lot more honest and open with patients than they used to be," Rossman believes. "In the past, they would say, 'Don't worry, I'll take care of all this, you're going to be okay.' They took all of the responsibility but they didn't always deliver. And I think medical school fostered that façade of knowing everything and never being wrong. Doctors tend to be more honest, sit by the bedside, display a sense of humor, and so on — that's really different from when I first started in nursing. Today's medical marketplace rewards team-oriented doctors rather than autocrats. Hospitals are bottom-line driven, so the organization will put up with a lot from doctors who bring in a lot of business. But they also value doctors who can develop and lead medical teams and deal with critical conversations in a sophisticated and professional manner. Nurses really appreciate this type of individual, too.

"Many hospitals are now taking a look at creating safer systems. Traditionally, one of the possible contributors to the problem of medical errors was that no one would question a physician because of his power, and they didn't want the backlash. In one scenario presented in a workshop on crucial conversations, we were told of a patient whose foot was amputated rather than given the tonsillectomy that he came to the hospital for. The authors of this scenario went around and back-tracked everyone who interfaced with that patient and found that there were no fewer than *seven* times when someone could have spoken up and said, 'Something is irregular here.' But no one did. In that atmosphere of 'we can't question orders' this kind of thing can happen. Now doctors are being sued, so this culture is changing, but it got this way because no one would question doctors."

Rossman stresses that we all have a stake in solving the problems of disruptive physician behavior.

"Effective doctor–nurse relationships have certain hallmarks: basic human respect, mutual respect, and an ability to communicate. Whether it's a cultural norm or a core personality disorder, when doctors are insulting, it has a negative impact on nurses. Nurses rank as number one on lists of professions that people view as being populated by people of integrity. It's important that hospitals and doctors support them so they can continue in that role."

The golden age of nurse–physician collaboration has yet to occur — the time where doctors and other members of their medical staff consistently combine their considerable talents in an atmosphere of patient-centered care and concern. Nevertheless, the United States is taking its first serious steps toward helping doctors learn to stand shoulder-to-shoulder with nurses and other medical colleagues, because experience has proven that when Doctor God becomes a team player, everyone wins.

CHAPTER 6
MANAGE ADVERSARIAL
RELATIONSHIPS

WHEN DOCTOR GOD goes on a rant, spouses and coworkers can suffer. No one, however, is more vulnerable to a doctor's attitudes and moods than those he has taken an oath to help: his patients.

When we get sick — regardless of the illness — all we want is to get well, and often that involves a visit to the doctor. The last thing we want is to be blown off as just another nuisance in the doctor's already hectic day.

I grew up with the idea that a doctor's word was law. His prescriptions were to be filled and taken, tests he ordered were to be undergone, and whatever he advised regarding my health and well-being was to be complied with. Period.

It never occurred to me that doctors were like me: living, breathing, fallible humans who rushed through their days making judgments on all manner of ailments, and it took me several years to begin questioning what they said.

I unfortunately suffered on many occasions the consequences of being the compliant and obedient patient, in the process experiencing some horrendous misdiagnoses (multiple sclerosis ranking near the top) and unnecessary procedures, such as sinus surgeries performed by a surgeon who used his patients' illnesses to procure drugs to support his own addiction.

PLEASE, JUST LISTEN TO ME!

Today's health-care industry is indeed hectic. Many doctors don't have the luxury of spending enough time with patients to get to know us, much less earn our respect. Appointments are rushed; part of the examination time is spent typing in notes on their laptops rather than listening to or talking with us about our health issues. Finally, with a flourish of the prescription pad, they're gone and we're left to wait for the nurse or medical assistant to finish up the appointment. If we are patients of a clinic or group practice, we might see a different doctor at each visit; if we're part of an HMO, we're likely to be referred to a series of specialists for even routine care or procedures. Caught in this factory-like approach to health care, many of us feel like nothing more than a doctor's source of income, rather than his or her partner in wellness.

No matter how bitter and critical a physician's ex-spouse may be following the irretrievable breakdown of their relationship, an ex-patient can be even angrier and more unforgiving. Most authorities — including doctors, psychologists, health-care administrators, insurers, and patient-advocacy groups — agree that the doctor–patient relationship is the most fundamentally important aspect of successful health care. We depend on our doctors to advise, treat, guide, and protect us. We rely on their training, knowledge, and judgment. We expect them to treat our well-being as a top priority, because we are forced to trust them with our lives.

Over the last thirty years or so, attitudes toward doctors have hardened. Some began to see them as wealth-seeking, authority-obsessed elitists — members of a profession who blithely ignore the needs and interests of the patients they are supposed to serve. On the other hand, doctors can harbor some pretty unkind ideas about patients, too, viewing them as ill-informed attention-seekers who won't follow instructions, who think that the latest article on "medschoolinaminute.com" makes them experts on their conditions, and who are just waiting for a doctor to slip up so they can sue for malpractice. The doctor–patient relationship also often tends to be more contractual than collaborative, and more adversarial than trusting.

One issue that fosters those attitudes is America's dissatisfaction with its health-care system. Our per capita spending for health care is nearly 2.5 times the median expenditure of countries in the rest of the industrialized world, yet we have less access to the benefits of that care — fewer doctors, fewer CT scanners, fewer MRI machines, and fewer hospital admissions per capita — than many other Western countries. The Institute of Medicine estimates that nearly eighteen thousand Americans die every year from heart attacks because they didn't get the preventive medication they were eligible for. More than half of all patients with some of today's most common and deadly diseases — diabetes, hypertension, congestive heart failure, asthma, depression, and chronic atrial fibrillation — are managed inadequately. At the same time, the number of deaths due to medical errors continues to rise.

Where do we patients lay much of the blame for these problems? Where do we direct the anger and frustration we feel when faced with the inadequacies of our incredibly expensive and often dysfunctional health care system? Much of the time, we blame our doctors.

If you're ever in need of a juicy conversation-starter that is guaranteed to stimulate the interest of even the most reclusive members of any social gathering, you can always fall back on this old favorite: "What's the worst experience you ever had with a doctor?" Try it sometime — but brace yourself for the verbal stampede you're likely to unleash. Many people can relate at least one story of medical arrogance, neglect, misdiagnosis, or malpractice in which they or someone they know was a victim. Here are just a few examples:

- A young woman developed intense migraines. Over months of failed treatment attempts, her doctor prescribed a series of drugs, including a frequently prescribed antidepressant. The woman continued to have migraines, though with less frequency. She also began gaining weight at an alarming rate, adding eighty-five pounds to her five-foot-two-inch frame within the period of only a few years. Her doctor chided her about her weight, sometimes to the point of being rude. The woman was so medicated that she wanted to do nothing but sleep; she missed work frequently and had little contact with friends or family. Then, the woman's husband was transferred, and the couple moved to a new state. The new doctor she saw there took her off most of the drugs, including the antidepressant. The woman saw no change in the frequency or patterns of her headaches, but she did begin to drop weight, losing almost fifty pounds within the first year. When her new doctor asked her what she was doing to lose weight, she said "nothing." He shrugged and said, "Must have been the [antidepressant]; it causes people to gain weight."

- After being released from the hospital following an emergency appendectomy, a fifty-eight-year-old woman developed a high fever, with swelling and redness at the site of her incision. For two days, her daughter called the attending doctor, who (when he returned her calls hours later) told her that her mother's reaction was "normal" and advised the daughter to continue giving her aspirins and plenty of water. The next morning, alarmed at her mother's rising temperature, the daughter took her mother to the emergency room. After a quick examination, the ER doctors determined that the mother's incision was infected. She went back into surgery, where her wound was surgically reopened, cleansed, and left open. For two weeks after her release, the daughter had to swab out and irrigate the open wound twice daily. Her mother later developed a large and irreparable hernia at the site, due to the incision being opened again so soon after the first surgery. The original doctor, rather than apologizing for his neglect and the problems it caused, told the daughter that "infections like that are common after emergency appendectomies."

- An elderly man was in an automobile accident and his doctor later called the man's wife and told her that her husband was going to have neurological problems. The doctor said that her husband couldn't remember anything about the accident, which had happened just a week before. But the patient's family quickly realized that the problem was that he didn't have his hearing aid in during his appointment and couldn't understand what the doctor was asking him. "We realized that we couldn't let him be alone with any doctors," the patient's son-in-law said, "because he had trouble communicating with them. That was truly frightening! We suddenly understood all those reports we keep hearing about how miscommunication is linked to the majority of cases in which people in hospitals die from medical errors."

- A seventy-eight-year-old woman developed heart arrhythmia, and her family doctor prescribed an anti-arrhythmia medication. The medication caused the patient to become dizzy and disoriented, so the GP recommended that she try taking a half dose. When the dizziness continued, he told the patient to stop taking the drug and see a cardiologist. After examining the patient, the cardiologist recommended that she go back on the same anti-arrhythmia drug, but at *double* the previous dosage. The patient told the cardiologist of her poor experience with the drug, and the doctor assured her that the problem was that she wasn't taking enough of it. "The dosage was about half what it should have been," he said. The patient again voiced her concerns, but the cardiologist dismissed them and assured her that her fears of the drug's negative effects were groundless. The patient reluctantly followed the cardiologist's recommendation, and within hours of resuming the medication, her blood pressure dropped dangerously low and she grew faint to the point of nearly losing consciousness. The woman was rushed to the emergency room and admitted to the hospital, where she spent the next few days in recovery. The cardiologist never apologized to the patient for failing to give credence to her concerns, or for the dangerous, expensive, and quite inconvenient outcome of his medical treatment plan. The doctor's sole comment about the incident was, "You never know with these things."

Manage Adversarial Relationships

Granted, these horrific individual incidents clearly don't represent the way every doctor interacts with patients. Nevertheless, we can say with some confidence that "broken" doctor–patient relationships are all too common.

Combine the medical training process itself that creates the aforementioned "medical personality" with the all-too-human frailties doctors bring into the profession with them — including personal prejudices that can interfere with their relationships with patients — and you have a recipe for trouble. As Sandeep Jauhar, MD, noted in an article he wrote for the *New York Times*: "Judgments about personality, character and worthiness are reflected in all aspects of the doctor–patient relationship, from the language doctors use to describe patients (hysterical, difficult, nice, solid) to the attitude we take into the examination room." Jauhar acknowledged that making judgment calls is part of a doctor's job; but he also wondered how often those judgments are moral, as well as medical. Although scientific studies are not needed to confirm that a doctor's prejudices can impact his or her ability to form effective working relationships with patients, Jauhar nonetheless cited some compelling findings from a review of recent research on the effects of doctor prejudice in health care:

- Blacks wait longer than do whites for kidney transplants (they even have to wait longer than whites to get on the waiting list) even though they suffer disproportionately from kidney failure.
- Women with heart disease receive fewer angiograms and catheterizations than do men, and are more likely to die from heart attacks and unstable angina; women with chest pain wait longer than do men for examinations in the emergency room.
- Doctors are more likely to withhold artificial ventilation, dialysis, and surgery from elderly patients than from younger patients — even when requests to withhold "extreme measures" are taken into account.

Rush to Judgment — Snap Diagnosis

In his groundbreaking book *How Doctors Think*, Jerome Groopman, MD, a researcher and professor at Harvard Medical School, reported on his own research into the ways doctor preconceptions and snap judgments can mold the doctor–patient experience and result in misdiagnoses and treatment errors. Groopman's own experiences and research lead him to conclude that doctors can, at times, use flawed thinking when evaluating patients and their illnesses. If a physician stereotypes patients according to their appearance, personality, or current situation, that physician can make what Groopman refers to as "attribution errors," where, for example, a middle-aged woman's severe headaches are attributed to menopause-induced migraines, rather than a fast-growing brain tumor. Even a physician's very human reaction to an individual can have disastrous results. "If the doctor doesn't like you," Groopman said in an interview with CBS news anchor Katie Couric, "he or she closes their mind off. It's a set-up for misdiagnosis."

Groopman also found that physicians can be guilty of quickly categorizing symptoms to arrive at snap diagnoses that aren't always accurate. If a doctor has seen a number of patients with the flu during the past few days and a new patient comes in with a fever and sore throat, the physician might quickly assume that that patient also has the flu, without asking questions to explore other possibilities. Rather than taking the time to listen to patients fully describe their symptoms or situation, says Groopman, doctors have been shown in studies to give patients an average of only eighteen seconds to speak before interrupting them — often with a fast-break diagnosis based on everything *but* the individual before them and the concerns that person is expressing.

There's just not much support in today's medical practice for a doctor–patient relationship based on strong communication, and that's a true shame. Multiple studies have confirmed what common sense suggests — that patients prefer doctors who speak with them as equals, who answer their questions, who listen and respond to their concerns, and who help them make their own informed health-care decisions. Strong communication results in a stronger doctor–patient relationship, which leads to greater patient satisfaction and cooperation and contributes to better medical outcomes. Under our current system of medical-care reimbursement, however, testing — not talking — pays the bills in most medical organizations. As one doctor's wife told me, "Most insurance companies pay a set amount for an appointment time or procedure. You're paid perhaps $115 whether you spend ten minutes or an hour with a patient. How long will you be in there? You figure it out."

According to a survey released by the Centers for Disease Control and Prevention in 2004, the mean time spent with physicians during office visits was just over 18 minutes. This figure includes visits with psychiatrists, which often are scheduled in one-hour blocks, but doesn't include the almost 5 percent of visits in which *no* doctor–patient contact took place. During a conversation about these statistics, one of our interviewees, a financial analyst with a well-known investment firm, said he thought that figure had to be wrong. "Eighteen minutes?" he scoffed. "I can't remember the last time I spent that much time with a doctor during an office visit."

Doctors seem to feel the crunch of shrinking face time with their patients, too; during our interviews for this book, multiple physicians bitterly confirmed that they typically can spend no more than ten minutes with each patient before they must move on to the next (making the eighteen-minute visit seem downright leisurely). Whatever the reality, the *perception* of being rushed through an office visit is widespread, and that means that many patients and their physicians don't feel that they have time to talk to each other. And there goes the relationship.

Many physicians today will tell you that patients are responsible for some of the problems that threaten the doctor–patient relationship. Patient loyalty, for example, has become a thing of the past — although that often is beyond the patient's control or desires. Many must seek health care where their HMO or insurance plan dictates. If a doctor drops off "the list," it may well signal the end of the relationship. The uninsured are even less likely to stick with a doctor out of loyalty. Money talks, and when it says, "You can't afford this much for health care," many feel forced to listen.

Nevertheless, because we live in an age where we can or must hop from doctor to doctor, we're in a much better position to compare the quality of treatment we receive among providers. We're evaluating our doctors now in ways we never have before. When they provide substandard care or treat us disrespectfully, most of us will speak up before moving on. At the same time, we need to accept more responsibility for the success or failure of our medical experiences. As we assume a more active role in our health care, we lose the luxury of idly shuffling through the medical system and blaming it and our doctors when we don't emerge at the other end in sterling health. Today, the best physician–patient relationships are partnerships, and smart patients and their families are active advocates for their own health-care needs.

PATIENTS' STORIES

Imagine having a chronic illness that drags on and on, leaving you with unanswered questions and even being totally ignored by the physician you're counting on to help you. Such were the experiences shared by Donna, Angie, and Lauren (all pseudonyms) in their encounters with the Doctor Gods from Hell. Their stories are not totally negative, however, because, with persistence and tenacity, they eventually hooked up with Doctors — not gods, but caring humans — from Heaven.

All of these women had happy outcomes, but their experiences are well worth reading and remembering.

Donna

As stated before, some women have problems working with doctors on pain management, particularly those suffering from migraines. One nurse told us, "I saw a doctor whose wife developed really bad migraines become very much more sympathetic to women patients reporting pain. Another one, on the other hand, was just the opposite. If a child had an earache or tonsillitis, he'd give them a light injection of Demerol for pain. But when it came to women, he would tell them to take Tylenol, look at his watch, and dismiss them."

In search of relief for migraines, Donna struggled through a five-year relationship with one neurologist but instead got over-medicated and a lack of respect from her doctor and his staff. Donna's story illustrates how difficult it can be to step up and demand better treatment when you are suffering from pain and living in a fog of pharmaceuticals. It also raises an often-asked question: Do doctors have a patient "blacklist"?

"I began seeing Dr. O because of my migraine headaches," Donna began. "I'd just moved to the area, and I'd been referred to him by my primary doctor near my old home. From the beginning, he was brusque with me. This neurologist never treated me like a person. He never talked to me about how I was doing or showed any interest in me or my overall health. All he talked about was my headaches. At every appointment he'd stare at his clipboard as he drilled me with questions like, 'How many headaches have you had since I last saw you? How do you rate them? How many of them made you throw up?' He prescribed a number of drugs for me — I think at one point I was taking five different medications — but the headaches weren't getting better, and I was dopey all the time.

"I continued to see my regular doctor as well, and he noted my continued problems with migraines and my general downslide under the effect of all those drugs. He gave me the name of another neurologist who was located very far away from my home and office. I was in so much pain and so foggy from all of those drugs, I couldn't bear the thought of starting over with another doctor."

In spite of everything, Donna continued to see Dr. O for four or five years. Prescriptions proved problematic.

"One of the drugs he prescribed was considered highly addictive," Donna said. "My prescription called for one bottle a week, and I could only pick up one bottle every Monday, which was fine most of the time. But if I had to be out of town or something, it was a real hassle to try to pick it up early. Usually, Dr. O's office reacted to me as though I was a dope fiend whenever I wanted the refill. And I kept saying to Dr. O, 'If you think this is bad for me, let's find something else. Let's use a different drug.' But he'd say, 'No, I think you need to use this one.'

"The blowup came when I had to go out of state to my son's wedding, which was going to be held at a rural retreat in the middle of Virginia. The event was going to last from Friday through Sunday, and I had to be at work really early on the following Monday. My drugstore doesn't open until nine in the morning, so I wanted to pick the drug up on Friday morning before we left for the wedding. I started calling his office early Thursday morning. They kept putting me on hold or saying he'd call me, but the office never called back. I was stressed out anyway, from preparing for my son's wedding. I finally left work to go home, and I called them on my way home. They put me on hold — again — so I just drove to his office. I was fed up. I went in and asked, 'Who's in charge of getting the prescriptions filled?' A woman came out from the back office and asked me what I wanted, and I told her in very specific terms that I was incredibly unhappy with their lack of response to my requests. The receptionist, who had no role in this issue at all, got upset and said I 'wagged my finger at her.'

"That seemed to start their ball rolling, and she and the other assistant started going off about how good they had always been to help me with my prescriptions. I said, 'Are you kidding? Call my pharmacist and ask how much time I've spent in the drugstore waiting on your office to call in a prescription, hours after it was originally requested.'

"I finally decided I had had it with this neurologist. I said, 'That's it. I've had other doctors tell me that your office is difficult to deal with, and you are. I should have found another neurologist long ago, and so this is just the impetus I needed to do that.' I walked out of that office for good. After this blowup, I knew that I had to get a new doctor. He had been rude and dismissive of me for years, and now I was getting the same kind of treatment from his receptionist!"

The response Donna got from Dr. O came shortly after her last visit in the form of a registered letter, which she didn't even open. She simply wrote "return to sender" and sent it back, thinking the issue over and done. That was, however, not the case.

"The next time I went to my regular doctor, the one who had first referred me to Dr. O," she said, "he was furious with me. He said, 'I'm never going to tell you anything again. You got me into big trouble with Dr. O,' and blah-blah-blah. He wasn't at all concerned with the fact that my condition wasn't better, that this doctor had put me on this long list of medications, then left me hanging when I needed prescription refills, or that his office workers had triggered a confrontation with me in the reception room. He was only concerned that I had said something that gave Dr. O the (correct) suspicion that he had said something uncomplimentary about him. It was obvious that the 'hot line' had been at work.

"After that, other doctors I went to seemed to have this attitude toward me, too. Not too long after, I had to go to the emergency room with a particularly bad migraine. The ER doctor was looking at my chart, and said, 'Well, maybe we need to have Dr. O give you a spinal tap.' What could that have been, other than some commentary on my confrontation with Dr. O? I couldn't help but think that there was some sort of black mark in my file, and that every other doctor who read it assumed that I was a problem patient and treated me as such. A short while later, I had an operation on my nose for a deviated septum and the nurse at the clinic said, 'Well, you *seem* like a nice person, but you never know.' I thought, *WHAT?* Why would she even say that to me? So I knew that one of my doctors had recorded something negative about me in my medical records. I felt as though I had been put on some sort of blacklist, at least in that area.

"In any event, I found another neurologist, one who practiced up near Baltimore. When I got in to see him, he said, 'I won't even take you on as a patient if you're going to take all of these drugs, especially this one (meaning the one Dr. O had given me so much grief about) — it's very dangerous.

"I said, 'I don't care whether I take any of them or not. They haven't done much good, so do whatever you think is best.' I couldn't help but remember that Dr. O had insisted I continue to take that drug, even after I told him he should switch it if it was such a 'danger.' And as far as it being habit-forming, I can't even remember what it was called now — so it wasn't like I was out on the street trying to score it."

Donna's new neurologist prescribed fewer, different drugs, and she feels much better.

"I have more energy, I feel healthier overall, and I have fewer headaches. The last time I saw him, he said I didn't need to see him again for a year, and if I was doing as well then as I am now, I could just see my regular doctor for updates on my prescriptions.

"So much for Dr. O — tie a bell to his tail! I really resented the way he and those in his office treated me. It was humiliating to go through that blow-up in his office. In retrospect, I am so glad it happened. I needed something to wake me up and get me out of that horrible treatment."

Angie

Switching doctors, even when you know you should, can be very difficult — especially when you are in the middle of a medical crisis. As Angie learned, though, working your way through a frightening medical experience can bring the clarity and strength one needs to insist on finding a doctor with whom you can forge a strong and effective working relationship.

As a teenager, Angie was diagnosed with neurofibromatosis, a relatively rare disorder of the nervous system that causes tumors to grow around the nerves. The first symptom of her disorder appeared years before the formal diagnosis, however, when Angie began suffering from crippling headaches. "I remember being six years old and having to go into a bathroom in a restaurant once, where I began throwing up from the pain of these headaches. I didn't know at the time that they were migraines, but that's what they were."

Angie's disorder was finally diagnosed at age fifteen. At that time, her doctor discovered some fatty deposits along some of the nerves in her neck, and recommended that Angie see a plastic surgeon for their removal, to avoid excessive scarring from the surgery. Unfortunately, no one, including the plastic surgeon, realized that these deposits actually were neurofibromas. He clipped them off and had them biopsied.

"That's when they realized I had neurofibromatosis," Angie explained.

For years, those migraines were the only ongoing symptoms of Angie's condition. As an adult, Angie found a primary care physician who was an area specialist in treating people with neurofibromatosis. Angie married, and for the next year and a half, enjoyed a happy, normal life with her new husband. She left her job as an assistant in a legal firm and took a job as a barista in a Starbucks kiosk in the lobby of one of the city's large hospitals. Despite the rosy appearance, though, her life didn't proceed happily ever after.

One morning in March of 2007 Angie got up as usual, dressed, and drove into work. She talked with her husband on her cell phone as she drove and felt fine. Then the hammer dropped.

"By the time I got into work," she said, "I felt as though my legs were going to come out from under me. I panicked. I knew where I was, but I had no idea what was wrong. I felt very weak and I was shaking. Someone asked if I was okay, and I couldn't find words or speak — I couldn't even describe what was happening to me.

"Someone at the hospital where I worked called my primary care physician, and she said to call the employee health department and have someone there take my blood pressure and temperature. But that office said they couldn't see me because technically I wasn't an employee. So they sent me to the ER in a wheelchair because I couldn't walk. The ER doctor was a friend of my primary care physician and called in a neurologist who happened to be at the hospital. After reviewing my condition, he recommended that I be admitted. They scheduled an MRI and scans and so on. The tests revealed nothing new, so they sent me home."

Angie's primary care physician didn't know what was going on or how to treat it. There was no treatment plan, no referral to other doctors or specialists who deal with people with long-term illnesses or chronic disorders. The doctor did nothing but prescribe different medicines, putting Angie on incredibly strong pain medication, which then constipated her, causing even more pain. Angie was then put on medication to counteract the constipation.

"I took that for two or three weeks," Angie recalled. "But I began vomiting every time I ate. My doctor said the new medicine was nauseating me, so she took me off that and switched me to another medication that suppressed my appetite, then also gave me medication to stimulate my appetite. I took anything because I assumed they knew what they were doing; they knew more than me. Looking back, I realize now that I was taking medications to counteract the effects of the medications they were giving me. I remember hearing one of the residents say to my physician, 'One of the contraindications of this drug is loss of appetite. Is this appropriate?' and my doctor dismissed the resident's concerns.

"By May, when there had been no change in my condition, my family and I realized we had to step in and insist on answers. I was still unable to eat and I was going downhill. My doctor thought there was something wrong with my mental state, like depression or something. She never said that to me, told me anything about that illness, or suggested any kind of psychotherapy or treatment for mental issues. She did say, 'If you don't start eating, I'm going to have to put you in the hospital and put in a feeding tube.' Of course, I had no appetite, to some degree because I was on medication that suppressed my appetite. And she was threatening me with hospitalization if I didn't eat!

"Both my husband and my father became very active at that point and continue to be so in monitoring what happens to me, doing their research, requesting specific tests and specialists. At their insistence we saw some other doctors — a cardiologist, a neurologist, a surgeon, a genetics doctor — because we pushed for them, not because my primary care physician recommended that I see them.

"The neurologist recommended further testing, and a PET scan revealed that I had tumors in my stomach. The genetics doctor found the fibroma on the PET scan, and we thought she'd saved my life. She's the one who seemed to be positive, the one who said, 'We're going to get this fixed.' She thought the tumors might be malignant. A surgeon removed the worst of them in July. It wasn't malignant, but the pain went away."

The surgery had gone well, but Angie still wasn't hungry, although she could eat some things. However, her pain medication was constipating her. The genetics doctor recommended going off the pain medication because it wasn't helping. They pulled her off the pain meds the Friday before Labor Day. By the following Tuesday, she was having serious trouble keeping food down. At first, yogurt and English muffins stayed with her, but within just a few weeks, even those came up.

"I called my primary care physician and told her something wasn't right," Angie said. "I went in to see her, and she put me in the hospital. The techs in the hospital couldn't get IVs started in my veins at first, because I was so dehydrated. After the fluids got into my system, I felt a bit better. They inserted a feeding tube and ordered that I have no food by mouth. Soon, I could get out of the hospital bed by myself and open the door, things I hadn't been able to do.

"My treatment in the hospital was alright. I had a wonderful nurse. He did small things that really mattered: He brought me gowns that actually fit, got me a hospital bed that was comfortable — things that might sound insignificant but were the saving grace. I learned that many nurses and techs will tell you about the procedures and equipment they're using if you ask them. You can really learn a lot about your treatment if you just pay attention and ask questions. My IV monitor flipped off a lot and started buzzing. I would ring for a nurse to come reset it, but usually I had to wait a long time, with that thing buzzing beside my head. I watched how the nurses reset the monitor, and if it went off, I'd reset it myself.

"But too often, no one is willing to listen to the patient — they treat you like you're an idiot. Once, while I was in the hospital, they took me down to have an endoscopy. I had a pick-line inserted in my arm, but they still had the IV in my wrist. I told the nurse, 'I have a pick-line, so I don't think you'll be able to get anything started in the IV.' And the nurse said, 'Don't worry about it,' and just went on preparing to start the IV. I said, 'Can you just call upstairs and ask my doctor about using the pick-line?' And she just ignored me and started talking about it to another nurse.

"I said, 'Excuse me — the patient is lying right here and I can hear everything you're saying. They haven't flushed this IV, so you won't be able to get it going. I really think you should call up and see about using the pick-line.' She said, 'I don't have time to call up there.' And I said, 'But you have time to stand here and argue with me?' So she began trying to push this solution through the IV and, sure enough, it wouldn't work. Finally, she called upstairs, and of course, was given permission to use the pick-line."

So there!

"I learned that I *had* to speak up more and try to manage my health care," Angie said ruefully. "I began asking questions about everything: 'What is that medicine you're giving me? Did you wash your hands?'

"My bathroom became so dirty that it smelled like a New York subway. I called the nurses in and told them they needed to get someone in to clean it. I became much more vocal. I asked questions about every test, every medication, every assumption about my health.

"I was released from the hospital almost three weeks ago, and it feels like things are under control. I can eat better, although I have this soft tissue mass that interferes with the processing of my food, so I have to take medicine to make the food move through my system. Being off of the pain meds has played a big role in making me feel better. Of course, it's been painful. The meds sedated my nerves, and now they're lively, tingling and sometimes giving me pain. That part is hard; I don't sleep well at night. But I know it's just the shock of my body returning to a nonmedicated state.

"I've seen a number of doctors and all of them have been trying to track down the specific cause of the problem. They believe that what happened was a complex migraine, which resulted in neuropathy in my legs. Because I haven't been able to eat normally since this started, they think now that it may have triggered something in my brain that turns off my hunger reflexes. Still, none of my doctors has been able to give me a definitive diagnosis. I think they still don't know what happened."

Angie now sees doctors and the health-care system in a very different light from how she did before.

"We were always taught to believe that doctors are the professionals, and we have to respect that. Now, I don't believe that my doctor is speaking the gospel. I've been seeing my primary care physician almost ten years. I thought we were on pretty good terms. I trusted her. But then, with this incident, I saw a real difference in her attitude. She might be a good doctor, but she couldn't say, 'I don't know what's going on. I can't figure this out, and I'm going to call someone else in.' Instead, it was just, 'Oh, you're back again, and you're still not eating, you're still not gaining weight. You need to start eating' — and this heavy sigh, as though she thought I was putting her through something, like I was a reminder that she had failed. I think she thought that if she didn't see me, she wouldn't have to think about it.

"So I don't think she wanted to see me."

As scared as Angie is of starting over with another doctor, she thinks she's likely to seek a new primary care physician.

"I'm definitely going to take an active role in my health care, no matter who I see," she said. "I'm not going to take prescriptions because someone says I should, and I'm going to ask lots of questions about any test I'm asked to submit to and the results of those tests. I realize now that I'm going to have to be the engine that drives my health."

Angie's new patient advocacy and activism carries through to all of her health care.

"I was at the dentist's office the other day. I have a latex allergy, which is stamped in bold red ink on my chart. The dental technician came in to start working on my teeth, and as she started toward me,

I saw that she was wearing latex gloves. I asked her if that's what they were, and she said, 'Yes, are you allergic?' I said yes, and she said, 'Well you should have said something earlier.' And I said, 'No, you should have read my chart.' So now, if the first words out of my mouth to dental technicians have to be 'I'm allergic to latex,' instead of 'Hi, how are you?' that's just the way it is."

Angie acknowledges it's not not easy being nice all the time. "Many people want to feel like they're friends with their doctor — or other professionals they deal with, for that matter," she said. "I was like that at one time. I thought, 'Oh, I want my doctor to think I'm funny or smart or whatever.' Then I realized, my doctor doesn't care! It's not going to benefit my health care, either. I was taught to respect people in authority and not question them. But now, I question everyone and everything.

"I've learned that the only professional you should be friends with is your bartender," Angie laughed, "because that's part of his job, and you want him to be nice to you when you come back."

Angie is still working at settling back into her life. "There are days when my outlook isn't good, and I have a hard time dealing with my health, emotionally. I know I can pass this on to my children if I ever have any, and that eats at me every single day. But overall, I have a better outlook on life. I feel stronger mentally, and I appreciate the small things: sitting down and eating dinner with my husband, cooking, talking on the phone with friends; being able to say 'Today is a good day: I got some sleep.'

"Just waking up is a good thing. I'm looking forward to driving again and becoming as independent as I used to be. I really believe this experience will end up making me stronger and more in control of my life than I have ever been."

Lauren

It goes without saying that the best time to take a proactive role in your health care management is *before* a medical disaster occurs. Lauren was a physically active college student when she began to realize things were not right with her body. The doctors she saw assured Lauren that she shouldn't worry about the results of tests they ran, but she refused to stop asking for answers to her concerns. Her instincts were right on; thanks to her persistent pursuit of information about her condition, Lauren was able to limit the damages caused by an autoimmune disorder called lupus. In the process, she has gained new respect for the importance of collaboration between doctors, as well as between doctors and patients.

"Let me start by telling you about how I got sick," she began. "I was diagnosed with lupus in November of 2005, but the road to that diagnosis started back in late 1999, around the time I was a sophomore in college. I donated blood for a blood drive, and got a letter back from the Red Cross saying I couldn't donate anymore because my blood showed a false positive for syphilis. The people at the Red Cross agency said don't worry about it, because it's just a false positive, and my primary-care physician also minimized it all to me. He said it happened to a lot of people and not to worry about it. But it bothered me, so I did some research of my own on the computer. Basically, I learned that my blood indicated that I could have an autoimmune issue. Through my research, I found out what labs [laboratory blood work] I should have done to check for possible problems associated with this false positive. Over a period of time, while going to my doctor for checkups and so on, I requested that specific labs be drawn. I felt like a hypochondriac, because I was pushing for such specific tests, but I really wanted answers. Eventually, the labs I'd asked for revealed definitively that I had a predisposition to lupus or rheumatoid arthritis and other autoimmune issues."

Through her research, Lauren learned that autoimmune disorders are incredibly hard to diagnose — also something no one told her. Again, her primary-care physician said not to worry, since she had no symptoms. For Lauren, that wasn't good enough.

"My doctor was tired of my questions," she said, "so he referred me to a hematologist. The hematologist said the same thing, but because this was a potential autoimmune issue, he referred me to a rheumatologist. This was in the summer of 2005. I went to a rheumatologist and got established with him. He reviewed my lab work and said, 'Well, you're established with me, even though you have no symptoms. If something comes up with you now, you are one of my patients.'"

Despite the rheumatologist's reassurances, as the weeks passed, Lauren's condition did not improve. "Between the summer and fall of 2005 I had very low energy and thought I had the flu. My stomach was giving me problems. The Saturday after Thanksgiving I came home and found that it was too painful to get out of bed. I was running a fever and my joints were just so inflamed that I couldn't move. The next Monday, I called my rheumatologist and said, 'I don't know what's wrong with me, but I can't move.' Because I was [already established as] his patient, I was able to get right in to see him."

The doctor suspected Lauren was having a first flare-up with lupus, so he ordered labs and prednisone [a steroid that would alleviate her inflammatory symptoms]. The lab results came back and showed she did indeed have lupus.

"It had taken me about three months to get into my first appointment with that rheumatologist, so thank goodness I had already established myself with him and could get an emergency appointment. There is a good chance that my primary care doctor wouldn't have known what was wrong with me. I went through a time when he was giving me diagnoses such as irritable bowel syndrome and chronic fatigue syndrome. I'm now a mental-health professional, and I see a lot of cases where anxiety creates and exacerbates physical conditions. I told my doctor I believed in those conditions, but also believed that they had underlying causes, whether emotional or physical. It took a lot of pushing on my part to come up with those answers. I don't think I was being blown off — I just don't think that the level of expertise was there to diagnose something as difficult as my condition. My own foresight and pushing was what made it possible for me to get timely treatment.

"I wasn't glad to get sick, but I was glad to have positive confirmation of what I really had."

Lauren discovered that she had to remain on top of her treatment and continue to work for a strong partnership with her doctors.

Manage Adversarial Relationships

"When I first got put on the steroids I responded very well. I could watch the clock and 'feel' myself feeling better. These are amazing drugs. My rheumatologist told me, 'When people first go on these drugs they want to hug me, but after a while, they want to punch me.' The side effects of these drugs are pretty dramatic. You gain weight, you're emotionally volatile, and you have sleep issues. So they do their job, but . . .

"About four days after I started taking the steroids I started having pain in my joints again, then pains in my chest, too. I went to the emergency room and found out that it was inflammation — the joints in my sternum were inflamed and causing the chest pain. But I had been scared that it was a problem with my heart, and I had many issues in terms of being in touch with my rheumatologist. His office was only open from 9 to 4, and closed for an hour at lunch. They were pretty bad about not answering the phone or returning messages — he didn't return any phone calls. It was frustrating and made me really angry. If you called at 3:45 with a question, you'd get put on hold then cut off. When you called back, the office was closed. The HMO I belonged to has four rheumatologists, two of whom are in the same practice, and the other two are an hour from my home."

Lauren felt that her options were very limited. She worked with her rheumatologist for six months, while getting sicker all the time. As it turned out, her fiancé's father is a general practitioner in the same health network as the rheumatologist, and is one of the people who refers to this doctor, so he thought he had some leverage with him. He called the rheumatologist and left a message saying, "Hey, this girl is sick and she needs some attention. She's not a complainer. You need to call her back and answer her questions."

"And he still didn't call me!" Lauren exclaimed. "I realized that he just wanted to hand out medication that would mask my symptoms. I didn't want my symptoms masked — I wanted my disorder treated. I experienced symptoms that he minimized and said, 'This is just part of your disease.' And I ended up being admitted to the hospital in April of '06. I was in there for four or five days, and they ran a series of tests trying to figure out what was wrong with me."

Lauren became even more frustrated because after she landed in the hospital, the rheumatologist became much more attentive.

"'This was caused by this or that,' and 'I told you about this in your last appointment,' she recalled. But no, she responded. "I never heard anything about this from you."

"Once I was discharged," she recalled, "he started calling me at home and regularly returning my calls. He probably was scared because he thought I was going to sue him. He knew I wasn't playing around, and he also knew there was another doctor who knew he hadn't responded to my calls."

For Lauren, the "partnership" was over.

"I wrote him a lengthy letter terminating my treatment with him, which I copied to my insurance company. I reminded him that he told me that lupus was a disease of momentum, and the longer it goes untreated, the more momentum it gathers. The longer he went without returning my calls or answering my questions, the more momentum my disease gathered and the worse it got. He didn't respond to my letter. We work on the same campus now; I saw him once but didn't speak to him. I just don't have a lot of positive things to say to or about him.

"I also did some research and found another rheumatologist who was outside of my health network. Because of my poor experience, I didn't have any problem getting authorization to go outside of the network. Most HMOs know that it's a lot cheaper to pay for appropriate care than to pay for emergency hospitalization. I [now] have to work with insurance companies a lot to obtain benefits for my clients; I know the words to say to the review boards, so I had no problem.

"It breaks my heart to think of the people who don't have my experience. I now work with several people in my practice who have family members with autoimmune issues, and I work with a lot of people who are low-income or low-education, so I know that people without the ability to deal with the system are really going to suffer."

Not only has Lauren benefited from a close working relationship with her doctors, her doctors collaborate closely with each other on her care. She got in to see what she describes as a really excellent rheumatologist, who then connected her with a neurologist because one of the effects of lupus was nerve damage in her legs and feet. The neurologist ended up following Lauren's care for more than a year, working with the rheumatologist, who then took on the bulk of her follow-up care. The physicians collaborated beautifully, which Lauren thinks is remarkable between two specialists.

The neurologist continues to take the "front seat," as Lauren puts it, likely because of the neurological issues that lupus patients face. "I went on a lot of steroids for a very long time, which is tough to do. They do their job, but they're terrible to be on. My neurologist was wonderful and understanding, and he said, 'I know it's awful to be on these medications, but the outcome will be worth it.' I was trying to make bargains with him almost daily at one point — 'If I go without symptoms for this many days, can I cut back on my medications?' and so on — but he kept me on the treatment dosage that he thought was right and helped me work through those times. He was always responsive to me, always returned my calls. I think that's worth noting, too, because he is the managing partner of one of the largest neurological centers in the state, so he doesn't have a lot of idle time. He is certainly very supportive of me. He's so well respected in the community, and he's not a young doctor — he has more years behind him than ahead of him. Yet, he's still so eager and open and willing to listen to his patients.

"Even his nurses were wonderful to me. When I was taking the steroids, I gained a lot of weight. We all have that 'scary weight'; one day I went in to see my doctor and I had reached it. I was so upset that I just sat down on the floor and cried. The nurse sat down beside me and put her arm around me and just stayed with me as I cried, telling me that I was going to be alright. She couldn't do anything about it, but she let me know that she cared and that meant so much to me. It encourages you to be compliant with treatment. They acknowledge that there *is* going to be bad stuff that goes along with this, but it *will* be worth it in the end — without minimizing the bad stuff that's happening."

Lauren's experience has changed the way she approaches all health-care provider–patient relationships — even those in her practice in which she's the provider. She believes she is a better listener now, taking what people have to say to her very seriously.

"My knee-jerk reaction might be to minimize something," she said. "But I don't do that so quickly now. I realize that I need to be mindful of the difficulties faced by someone who isn't as articulate or able to express their needs or issues as clearly as a highly educated person might be. Overall, my experience has encouraged me to be more assertive.

"Because I had to be."

Furthermore, Lauren now regularly encourages others to press for answers to their medical concerns.

"Maybe I'm just a worrier by nature. It worried me that I had this thing, that I didn't know what it was or where it came from. In retrospect, it seems proactive, but at the time I was just scared and I needed an answer. And I wasn't satisfied with 'don't worry about it.' I'm not one to do what I'm told. That that's one thing that really gets people in trouble, being complacent and accepting what somebody tells you. We all need to do research and become our own advocate. I would be *very* sick right now if I hadn't been my own advocate. A year ago at this time I couldn't walk right, and now I go running. The recovery has been quite dramatic, and it wouldn't have been if I hadn't acted.

"I'm not happy to have lupus, but it's made me a stronger person. It's also made me a healthier person, which might seem strange. For my health insurance, you have to get your weight, cholesterol, and blood pressure measured; the better your results, the less money you have to pay toward your health insurance. When I was tested a year after my diagnosis, my insurance ended up costing much less, even though I was sick, because my illness had forced me to take better care of my health. I was eating better and exercising — doing the things we're all supposed to do, but I had a very strong motivation to do it. This isn't about looking good; now, it's about being healthy.

"Whether it has to do with your finances, health, or whatever —

when it comes to taking care of or looking out for yourself or your family, you have to step up and take responsibility. Of course, there's a fine line between assertive and aggressive. We want people to like us. But I have to remind myself that as much as I've been blessed to have people caring for me who are also very kind and likeable, I don't go to a doctor to make friends. If I have questions and they're not being answered, I push to make sure I get those answers. I know my doctors' schedules are tight and their time is limited. I write down my questions before I go in so I don't forget something important and we can stay on track. My neurologist and I have a great relationship now. I go in and I say, 'Dr. J, look what I can do. You know, for a while, I couldn't walk straight, and now I can stand on my toes.' And when I say, 'Look what you've done for me!' he always puts it back on me and says, 'No, you've done this for yourself.'

"I think it's important to remember there are really good doctors out there who don't have big heads or big egos, and it's important for them to be complimented for their good work. My doctor is very humble; he's been absolutely wonderful. Of course, there are doctors out there who aren't competent. If you run across one, find another. Don't be stopped by your HMO, either. You just have to find a good reason why it's medically necessary for you to see someone outside your network."

Lauren acknowledges that she has leapt a big hurdle, probably one of the biggest she will face in her life. She also understands that she will encounter other problems, but she faces that future with an enhanced self-assurance.

"I know now how to be my own advocate," she said, "and that I need to be knowledgeable about my own condition."

CHAPTER 7
CONSIDER THE ALTERNATIVES

ONLY A FEW YEARS AGO, it was completely the responsibility of our doctors to tell us what to do regarding heath care, when to do it, and, if necessary, in which hospital it would be done. We trusted them implicitly. Besides, who were we to even consider questioning their judgment?

YOU HAVE CHOICES!

What a different medical world we live in today. Not only do we question everything the docs tell us, but we in turn tell *them* what *we* have decided to do. If a recommended surgery is costly, we're hot on the Internet investigating every option; then we decide which hospital (whether in this country or overseas) offers the most bang for our medical bucks for the procedure.

Aside from surgeries, we have other health-care choices. For instance, we may elect to become an annual dues-paying member of a small medical service operated by one or two doctors who have declared independence from insurance companies and their accompanying time and reimbursement constraints. Imagine being able to call your doctor and actually not only be able to talk to him or her any time of the day or night, but maybe even have that physician make a house call! Such practices are expensive, of course, and not in the price range of everyone, but they often offer a menu of personal services that appeal to busy, affluent patients.

Also, the array of hospitals, specialty clinics, and surgery centers has greatly expanded in the past twenty years. Posh boutique-type hospitals appear more like luxury hotels than medical facilities and certainly seem like they would be more restful than the large, corporate hospitals.

A multitude of selections is available also if wellness is your concern. Traditionally, physicians were trained to deal with healing: writing prescriptions, performing surgery, and offering advice about ailments. Today, many doctors are focusing more on preventive practices and working with their patients to keep illness at bay.

Wellness advice can come from many sources other than doctors, however, including complementary and alternative medicine (CAM), specialists, nutritionists, Internet research, and a host of other possibilities. Patients have more power than ever before and are discovering that finding what's right for them and exercising their options are the keys to better health and optimum well-being.

TAKING A TRIP FOR YOUR HEALTH CARE

In 2006, West Virginia lawmaker Ray Canterbury made national headlines when he introduced House Bill 43596, which would allow enrollees in the state government's health plan to travel to foreign countries for surgery and other medical services. In fact, not only would the bill allow for such a choice, it encourages it; those choosing to go to an approved foreign clinic for a procedure covered by the plan would have all of their medical and travel expenses (including those of one companion) paid, plus be given 20 percent of the savings they racked up by having the procedure done overseas, rather than here at home.

Canterbury's bill drew attention to a growing international boom in medical tourism — an industry with special appeal for many of America's 61 million uninsured or underinsured citizens. At prices as much as 80 percent to 90 percent lower than those here in the States, hospitals in countries such as Costa Rica, Thailand, India, and the Philippines offer a wide range of health-care procedures in accommodations equal to or even better than their American counterparts. Some sources estimate that a half-million Americans went overseas for medical treatment in 2006 alone, and that it could become a $40 billion industry by 2010.

According to Canterbury and other proponents of medical-service outsourcing, the idea is all about competition; furthermore, they believe the rate of health-care inflation in this country — at almost four times the rate of overall inflation — has placed an unsustainable burden on the American economy.

"The best way to solve this problem is to rely on market forces," Canterbury writes. "My bills are designed to force domestic health-care companies to compete for our business."

It's hard to argue with the economics of medical outsourcing. According to MedicalTourism.com, the cost of typical heart bypass surgery in the United States is $130,000. The same operation is estimated to cost approximately $10,000 in India, $11,000 in Thailand, and $18,500 in Singapore. A $43,000 hip replacement in an American hospital costs $9,000 in India, or $12,000 in either Thailand or Singapore. Even adding the costs of travel and lodging, consumers stand to save real money by traveling overseas for these and many other types of routine surgery, including angioplasties, knee replacements, and hysterectomies.

Of course, many people have serious concerns about the idea of shopping overseas for invasive medical procedures. What about the quality of the service? What about follow-up care? And what happens if something goes terribly wrong? Those backing the business — including employers and lawmakers who are desperately seeking ways to cut the cost of employer-sponsored medical care — are quick to answer these concerns.

Most of the foreign medical facilities courting Western tourists are state-of-the-art, offering luxurious accommodations and individual around-the-clock nursing attention. Thailand's Bumrungrad Hospital, for example, offers five-star-hotel-quality rooms, a lobby that includes Starbucks and restaurants, valet parking, an international staff and interpreters, a travel agent, visa desk, and a meet-and-greet service at Bangkok's Suvarnabhumi Airport. In a 2007 report broadcast on NPR, an American woman said that when her doctor in Alaska announced that she needed a double knee replacement at a cost of $100,000, she replied that she couldn't afford the treatment. Her doctor recommended that she wait four years, when she would be eligible for Medicare. Instead, the woman opted for treatment at Bumrungrad, where the two knees were replaced at a cost of $20,000 (including the services of two physicians, an anesthesiologist, and physical therapy), and she was able to recover in the hospital's luxurious surroundings with her husband at her side. Her husband, who had undergone surgery in the United States the previous year, couldn't believe the amount of attention his wife received from her doctors and nurses, whom he said were in almost constant attendance.

Why is all of this lavish treatment and high-quality care so much cheaper abroad than it is here? We need only to look at all of the other services the United States has outsourced in the past decade to find the first part of the answer to that question: In places like Thailand and India — two popular destinations for cardiac, orthopedic, and cosmetic surgery — salaries are much lower than in the United States. Further, most services are provided under one roof, and patients select and pay for their medical services up front — no insurance billing. Medical malpractice liability insurance and claims caps in some foreign countries also help keep costs down.

What about the safety of foreign medical facilities? Bumrungrad Hospital is accredited by the Joint Commission International (JCI), the same organization that accredits U.S. hospitals, and has over two hundred U.S. board-certified physicians. That hospital isn't unique in the world of international medicine. Increasing numbers of medical tourism facilities are staffed by American and European-trained physicians and backed by well funded research facilities. Dubai, already a luxury travel destination, is preparing to enter the business of international medical practice and research in a very serious way. The 4.1-million-square-foot Dubai Healthcare City, slated to open in 2010, will offer academic medical research facilities, disease treatment, and wellness services backed by the oversight of a number of international partners, including a new department of the Harvard School of Medicine.

Most baby boomers love to travel and many of them are only too happy to combine foreign travel experiences with low-cost and high-value medical procedures. Furthermore, many insurance companies are also eyeing medical outsourcing as a way to cut costs for both enrollees and their employers. Blue Cross/Blue Shield of South Carolina, for example, is working with Bumrungrad to provide overseas alternatives for health care to its members.

Of course, one or two horrific medical mishaps alone could seriously damage the medical tourism industry. Most foreign countries don't support malpractice litigation to the extent that we do here in the United States, and fears of the "what-ifs" are keeping many private individuals and organizations from plunging in until they have a few more years to observe the medical outsourcing industry in action. For now, however, foreign medical facilities are anxious to maintain standards high enough to avoid any claims of malpractice, and many Americans, with their fondness for bargains and luxury, are more than willing to give those facilities an opportunity to prove their worth.

As good as medical tourism may be for us patients, it could have nasty overtones for America's already ailing hospital system. If patients travel to foreign lands to avoid pricey surgeries here at home, what kind of financial hit will American hospitals face? At 2007's International Medical Tourism Conference in Las Vegas, hospital physicians and administrators from around the globe gathered to discuss the issues surrounding medical tourism and their impact on the health care industry. In an interview about the conference, Sparrow Mahoney, chief executive officer of Medical Tourism and conference co-chair, admitted that American medical facilities are now in direct competition with their foreign competitors. "Hospitals will feel a pinch," she said.

BOUTIQUE PHYSICIAN PRACTICES AND FACILITIES

Most of us have had the frustrating and sometimes frightening experience of waiting for medical care we desperately need. We have a raging fever and are told that the doctor can see us in three days. If we choose instead to go to the emergency room of a nearby hospital, we may wait for hours in a roomful of equally ill and distressed people, their impatient spouses, parents, or screaming children, and constantly chiming cell phones. If our doctor agrees to "work us in," we're faced with an only slightly less daunting process, requiring a wait of what might be an hour or so. When we finally get before a doctor, we're rushed through a few minutes of evaluation, given a prescription, and sent on our way — typically worn out and much worse for the wear of the experience.

But many Americans are opting out of this tribal experience, and choosing instead to pay an annual fee (typically $3,000 to $30,000 above insurance costs) to retain the personalized, private care of a family physician. The "boutique" health-care movement began in the early 1990s in Seattle, Washington, and has since spread to urban areas around the nation. Instead of waiting days, weeks, or even months for an appointment that fits a doctor's schedule, members of these plans schedule medical visits at *their* convenience.

Need a house call? Not a problem with most boutique or "concierge" plans; members have their doctor's cell phone number and can simply call to arrange for the doctor to come to their homes. If a plan member needs to see a specialist or go the emergency room, he or she is accompanied by a plan physician.

There's no more rushing through appointments, either. While many primary care physicians juggle caseloads of as many as three thousand or five thousand patients, doctors in boutique plans might have no more than a few hundred patients under their care; Seattle retainer medicine pioneer MD^2 (pronounced "MD Squared") limits its doctor loads to no greater than fifty patients.

Some retainer plans require that members also carry insurance, while others refuse to process insurance payments at all. In a 2005 report on boutique medicine by CBS 5 News in northern California, one doctor complained that he had lost patience with insurance companies that require reams of tedious paperwork and billing regulations, then reimburse at 20 percent of his billing rate. "I went to medical school to be a doctor and take care of patients," says Jordan Shlain, MD, of the San Francisco group On Call. "I didn't take one class on billings, on insurance company shenanigans, or on the HMO grip."

Although some concierge medical services charge fees aimed squarely at the middle class, most admit that their fees put them out of the range of many people. Indianapolis' FirstLine Personal Health Care charges members an annual retainer of a few thousand dollars in return for twenty-four-hour access to one of the plan's doctors, unlimited office visits, and a small USB "key-chain" hard drive loaded with their medical records. Even though their fees are modest in comparison with some concierge medical services, FirstLine doctors Kevin McCallum and Timothy Story know that many of the patients they saw prior to forming the service are unable to afford membership. McCallum acknowledged in the *Indianapolis Business Journal* that FirstLine's fees would make his services unaffordable for some patients he's seen for twenty-five years.

Kevin McCallum was my primary physician for several years until his switch to "specialized care" led me to search for a different doctor. Although I am in my mid-seventies, I'm fortunate to be very healthy and take very few prescription drugs. Whether or not I could afford his services was beside the point: I don't feel the need for this kind of medical "hand holding."

Like other doctors around the country, however, McCallum and Story believe that retainer medicine offers the only option for family medicine doctors trying to escape the grinding demands of escalating practice costs and patient case loads. With many family physicians around the country retiring early and many medical students avoiding the low pay and high demands of a typical family practice, retainer-fee medical groups might be the most viable way to keep the "good old family doctor" in business.

We have yet to see what will happen when the average American is financially excluded from most family medicine clinics and groups — a fate that may occur in the not-so-distant future. Kevin Grumbach, MD, of the University of California at San Francisco, was in family practice for over twenty years and now worries that the rush to boutique medical services is threatening our nation's system of medical care. "I have grave concerns," he told a CBS 5 news reporter, "that . . . we are as a profession abandoning the need of the vast majority of Americans, . . . middle-class people who are increasingly left behind in an increasingly inequitable system."

Family medicine groups aren't the only specialty medical services spreading throughout the nation. An increasing number of small, doctor-owned hospitals and clinics (boutiques) cropped up over the past several years, most catering to niche markets of services in the lucrative medical areas of "hearts, brains, and bones" (cardiovascular care, orthopedics, and neurosurgery). These clinics tend to be extremely profitable. They attract physicians who feel that by establishing a specialty clinic they can increase both their income and their professional autonomy.

Because of the limited scope of services these clinics offer, they can keep their staff and operating costs much lower than those of general hospitals. As a result, even middle-class patients with insurance can take advantage of the private rooms, gourmet meals, pre-bedtime massages, and other perks available at some specialized facilities. Those that don't offer especially luxurious surroundings compensate by charging well below most general hospitals — reduced rates that make them popular with insurers. Furthermore, because of their smaller size and more individualized services, most boutiques boast a high medical success rate, too; stay rates for many procedures are lower than those of general hospitals, as are complication and mortality rates.

The majority of medical policy analysts agree, however, that boutique hospitals aren't the cure for our nation's health care woes.

By bleeding off the most profitable types of medical procedures, boutique hospitals drastically diminish the profitability of larger hospitals. In 2003, Congress temporarily called a moratorium on the construction of new specialty clinics, in response to fears that they were badly eroding the profits of full-service hospitals. The ban ended in 2005. According to Reed Abelson reporting in the *New York Times*, in just two years after the ban was lifted, the number of these facilities in the United States increased by 40 percent.

The news for patients isn't all good, either. In that same article, Abelson reported on two cases in which patients at small, doctor-owned specialty hospitals died from post-surgical complications and no physician was present to help them. In both cases, the staff of the smaller hospitals dialed 911 to get help for the patients; one patient was transported to a nearby general hospital where doctors pronounced him dead. In the wake of these incidents, Medicare began reviewing its policies to determine how these hospitals should be regulated.

Once more, patients are left to weigh the costs and benefits of specialty medical services. No boutique hospital will handle the wide variety of medical problems humans present on a daily basis — car crash injuries, gunshot wounds, infectious diseases, and other calamities typically require the diverse medical services provided by a community clinic or hospital. None of us wants to live in an area where the nearest all-purpose general hospital (and its ever-important emergency room) has been driven out of business by a local boutique clinic. And most of us would be uncomfortable undergoing surgery at a facility that might be left dialing 911 in a pinch. Nevertheless, these facilities are here to stay, and they offer one more option when choosing our own health-care solutions.

CAM — Consumer and Alternative Medicine

Have you ever taken Vitamin C to help combat a cold? Have you used deep-breathing exercises to fight off anxiety or pain? Are you a vegetarian, or do you follow the Pritikin, Atkins, or Ornish diets? If so, you've ventured into the world of complementary and alternative medicine (CAM). Although many of us were taught to think of alternative medicine as little more than quackery based on the superstitions and ignorance of its gullible believers, millions of Americans today will confidently state that this attitude itself is a product of ignorance.

For most of the past century, Western schools of medicine adhered strictly to the teaching of evidence-based medicine — medical science founded on the results of experimentation, testing, and scientific observation. However, in the centuries preceding the "scientific method" and the absolute identification of diseases, we sought wellness, which includes the treatment of illness as well as disease, through a number of CAM practices: meditation, massage, yoga, acupuncture, prayer, and many other ancient techniques for healing body and mind.

Our knowledge of science, physics, biology, and the workings of the human body has grown exponentially along with our understanding of illness and disease, but the techniques of many alternative health practices remain relatively unchanged since first recorded — and probably even before.

Our attitudes toward these practices, however, have undergone dramatic shifts over the years. In the past few centuries, every medical advancement has pushed the ancient healing traditions further into the background of our human experience. Traditionally, conventional doctors — those holding an MD or DO (doctor of osteopathy) — were dismissive or even derisive about nontraditional, alternative therapies. Many patients who approached their doctor with questions about the benefits of meditation, homeopathy, herbal therapies, or Chinese medicine, met a brick wall of resistance.

That is no longer the case overall, and we are seeing what once was considered strictly alternative medicine become mainstream. First, CAM is attractive to a diverse group of individuals, which makes it big business. According to a 2002 study that surveyed tens of thousands of Americans about their health-care activities and experiences, nearly 40 percent of the respondents used some form of CAM within the preceding year. When the survey specified megavitamins and prayer as health-related therapies, the figure rose to over 60 percent, and nearly 75 percent had used CAM at some time in their lives. Women were more likely than men to use CAM, as were people with a higher education, and those with a recent hospitalization. Former smokers also were more likely to use these therapies than current smokers or those who have never smoked.

Mind–body medicine was the most commonly used category of CAM; nearly 53 percent of those surveyed said they had used that, as opposed to only 0.5 percent reporting the use of energy-based CAM therapies. Prayer (both for self and others) was the most common specific therapy used, followed in order by natural products, deep breathing, meditation, chiropractic, yoga, massage, and diets. Most people used CAM because they thought it would help their condition if used in combination with conventional medicine; about half said they tried it because they thought it would be an interesting experience. A much smaller percentage reported that they had turned to these therapies because they thought conventional medicine would not help their condition or was too expensive.

Excluding the use of megavitamins and prayer for health maintenance, the most common reasons for using CAM therapies centered on pain management — back pain, neck pain, joint pain, arthritis, headache, and recurring pain. Surprisingly, though, the common head cold was the second-highest reported condition that prompted people to turn to CAM. Anxiety and depression, stomach upset, and insomnia also made the list.

The 2002 survey didn't ask what respondents spent on CAM, but figures from a 1997 national survey found in that year alone Americans spent between $36 billion and $47 billion on CAM therapies. Between $12 billion and $20 billion of that money came directly out of individual pockets rather than from insurance-covered services, which is more money than we paid for out-of-pocket expenses associated with all hospitalizations that year. Five billion dollars went to herbal products alone, and it's probably safe to assume that number has ratcheted up dramatically in the ten years since.

Consider the Alternatives

The shifting attitudes toward CAM are evident even in the terms we use to describe those therapies. Over the past few decades, practices referred to as "holistic" or "alternative" medicine by proponents, were just as likely labeled as "unconventional," "unproven," or "irregular" medicine by skeptics eager to emphasize that the techniques were scientifically untested and unproven.

In 1999, recognizing the growing acceptance and importance of complementary and alternative therapies, the federal government launched the National Center for Complementary and Alternative Medicine (NCCAM), a research arm within the National Institutes of Health.

According to NCCAM, complementary medicine includes unconventional therapies used in conjunction *with* conventional medical approaches, such as combining acupuncture with physical therapy to reduce joint pain. The term "alternative" medicine is applied when unconventional therapies are used *in place of* conventional medicine, as in substituting herbal therapy for hormone therapy to treat symptoms of menopause.

Using rigorous scientific methods, NCCAM demonstrated proven evidence of safety and health benefits for some CAM therapies, which are used in conjunction with conventional medical techniques in *integrative medicine*, a third category of medical treatment. As the organization continues to test alternative therapies, those approved move into the realm of conventional medicine.

Those broad definitions take in a vast collection of health-care approaches, practices, systems, and products that fall outside the current boundaries of conventional Western or mainstream medicine. NCCAM, however, groups all alternative therapies into one of five categories:

- *Alternative medical systems* are principles, practices, and theories that form a complete approach to medical care; traditional Chinese medicine, Ayurveda, homeopathy, and naturopathy are examples of these systems.
- *Mind–body interventions* make use of the mind's ability

to influence the body's physical condition and functions, including meditation, prayer, hypnosis, dance, and art therapies. You might have used a mind–body intervention program without even realizing it: patient support groups and cognitive–behavioral therapy, for example, used to be in this category of alternative approaches to mental health therapy but are now considered mainstream medical practices.

- *Biologically based therapies* use natural substances such as herbs, nutraceuticals (nutritional supplements), food, and vitamins to treat symptoms and promote health.
- *Manipulative and Body-based therapies* involve moving and manipulating one or more parts of the body to reduce symptoms and improve wellness; examples include massage, chiropractic, and osteopathic treatments.
- *Energy therapies* are treatments based upon the use of energy fields and include two types: *biofield* therapies, such as qigong, Reiki, and Therapeutic Touch, are designed to manipulate energy fields that surround the human body; *bioelectromagnetic–based therapies* involve the therapeutic use of electromagnetic fields.

Dale Guyer, MD, received training in both conventional and alternative forms of medicine. A graduate of the Indiana University School of Medicine, where he completed his residency in 1994, Guyer is now Medical Director of the Guyer Molecular Institute in Indianapolis. The facility's practitioners come from a number of medical disciplines, including Asian medicine and naturopathy. The overall medical approach is a holistic one that incorporates treatments designed to promote both mind and body wellness.

Although the overall climate in the medical community and society in general is more receptive to alternative treatments, Guyer concedes that many are still reluctant to get on board. "Doctors who are part of the old guard tend to adhere to the concepts and ideas taught to them in their schooling," he said. "They're not motivated to step beyond that training unless they have some personal experience."

That "old guard" seems to be on its way out, though. "Like the dinosaur, [the Doctor God personality] has had its day. Entry strategies for medical school are starting to improve that situation as well. With a more equal balance of gender in the medical workforce, we can expect to have more intuitive, caring contributions." Guyer sees the changing attitudes of doctors as being the result of those changes within the student selections at medical schools. "Today," he said, "half of the people entering medical school come from divergent backgrounds — theater, art, dance, and religious studies."

But when you get right down to it, we can thank the old-time paternalistic, autocratic Doctor God and the managed-care movement in part for the rising influence and availability of alternative medicine in the United States. During the past few decades, as health-care costs grew and Americans became impatient with the lack of time and personalized attention received from physicians, more people explored alternative medical therapies. During the 1990s, public acceptance of CAM surged, and the interests of government and the private sector weren't far behind.

In a 2002 interview for the *FRONTLINE* documentary "The Alternative Fix," James Whorton, MD, professor of Medical History at the University of Washington, spoke about why he believed American interest in CAM developed so rapidly. The dwindling time allotted to patients in most traditional physician practices ranks high on the list. Because most alternative practitioners don't answer to insurance company pay schedules or managed care treatment guidelines, they can spend much more time talking with patients, listening to their concerns.

"They also [tend to] pay more interest to the patient's personal subjective experience of the illness," said Whorton, "and not be quite so fixated on what the organic pathology is." In other words, we patients don't want to be classified by our condition, but rather known, understood, and evaluated as individual human beings."

Whorton further noted that advancements in traditional medicine also contributed in the push toward alternatives. Medicine racked up an impressive set of public-health programs, preventive treatments, and antibiotic cures for infectious diseases during the mid-twentieth century. Yet, as those diseases faded from the scene, we were left facing much more difficult-to-manage chronic diseases such as diabetes, cancer, and heart disease. Right now, we have no cures for these conditions, so we have to learn how to manage them. The majority of traditional doctors simply aren't trained as well for that aspect of medicine; if they can't fix a medical problem, they have little to offer patients who need to know how to find the best way to live with it. Many alternative therapies strive to do just that.

Marcia Angell, MD, a senior lecturer at Harvard Medical School, is no cheerleader for complementary and alternative medicine, but she agrees that Americans have turned to those therapies out of frustration with the managed care movement and other drawbacks of mainstream medicine at the end of the twentieth century. In "The Alternative Fix," Angell told interviewers, "While medicine has grown more and more powerful, scientific medicine — the means for delivering it — has become less and less satisfactory."

In short, CAM is big business in this country. Doctors, HMOs, hospitals, clinics, and other health-service providers, who at one time staunchly dismissed the benefits of alternative therapies, now include complementary treatments in their practices. Furthermore, CAM techniques and background studies are now included on the curriculum of many medical training programs. Pharmacists, nurses, and doctors are learning about CAM during basic training, rather than being encouraged to treat these therapies as some sort of weird departure from "real" medicine.

A 2002 survey of more than 700 doctors in Colorado inquired about their attitudes toward the use of CAM in their practices or among their patients. Fewer than half (about 300) responded, but of those almost 60 percent said their patients had asked about alternative therapies; that same percentage of doctors said they wanted more information about alternative therapies so they could discuss them with their patients. Interestingly, 24 percent of the doctors personally used alternative therapies, and that figure corresponded with the physicians' likelihood of bringing up the subject of CAM with their patients. Only 8 percent asked their patients about alternative therapies *every* time, and about 17 percent never asked. While 44 percent reported a somewhat or very positive attitude toward alternative therapy, 40 percent were neutral on the subject, and only 16 percent had a somewhat or very negative attitude.

Make no mistake about it — the two facets of medicine aren't melding into one. But more doctors and medical staff understand the benefits of integrating CAM therapies into conventional treatment practices. According to the National Academy of Science, cancer treatment centers are among the most common sites for integrative approaches to treatment. The Integrative Medicine Service of the Memorial Sloan–Kettering Cancer Center, for example, uses mind–body therapies, music, massage, and reflexology to treat cancer patients. Many conventional doctors also incorporate CAM into their treatment plans by referring patients to acupuncturists, for example, or massage therapists for supplemental pain or symptom management.

Once again, we patients are the ones driving this cozier relationship between alternative therapies and traditional medicine. When asked to defend the Beth Israel Medical Center of New York's decision to add homeopathy and other alternative therapies to their treatment roster, former president and CEO Matt Fink, also appearing on the *FRONTLINE* documentary, said it was simply a matter of meeting the demands of patients. Hospitals that don't offer those programs, he added, will see their patients go elsewhere. "My personal view of homeopathy is I don't understand how it works," Fink said, "and I'm not personally convinced that it does work. But that doesn't mean that I would prevent a homeopathy practitioner from working here." After all, lost patients equal lost revenue, an equation few hospitals can live with today.

Nevertheless, some health-care educators and analysts fear that a growing market for alternative treatment is driving the rising interest at medical schools and hospitals in teaching and embracing the practices. Harvard's Marcia Angell cautions that medical schools need to teach about the evidence that supports alternative and complementary therapies, rather than just promoting them as the next best thing in medicine — or, as she phrases it, "pandering to the market."

The controversy about alternative practices rages on, even as it becomes more acceptable in the world of mainstream medicine. Most experts agree that we need to do even more to educate both conventional and CAM practitioners about the benefits of the two approaches to medicine. Remember, not all CAM therapies are considered safe — let alone effective — by all doctors.

Patients also need to become more knowledgeable about the use of complementary and alternative medicines and practices. We frequently hear the warning that just because something is "natural" doesn't necessarily mean that it's "safe" under all uses and conditions, but too many of us fail to heed the advice. While research has shown that most of us use alternative therapies in combination with conventional medical treatments, unfortunately, a majority don't reveal that important detail to their conventional doctor — which can lead to some very unpleasant outcomes. In fact, we don't even *know* how dangerous it can be. Mixing herbal supplements with prescription medications can lead to side effects that haven't even been documented. For example, St. John's Wort can potentially interfere with the effectiveness of drugs used to prevent organ transplant rejection and others used to treat AIDS.

We take a huge leap of faith when we believe in the ingredients list on a bottle of herbal supplements. Manufacturers' claims on these products aren't verified by the FDA, and according to NCCAM, published analyses have found differences between what the bottle claims to contain and what's actually in there. NCCAM's website warns, "Some herbal supplements have been found to be contaminated with metals, unlabeled prescription drugs, microorganisms, or other substances." Further, as natural products, herbs vary in potency, and we can overdose on them just as we can on pharmaceuticals.

Consider the Alternatives

In the end, education is the key on the part of both patients and physicians. Dale Guyer summed it up: "Every day you have to be willing to know that you are so far away from knowing everything. I ask every day that I be open-minded because you can't know it all. If you really care and want to continue to progress, you have to keep learning."

CHAPTER 8
CREATE YOUR OWN
HEALTH PROGRAM

DOCTORS TODAY ARE caught in an era of conflicting goals and shifting professional realities. And their struggle to align themselves with those changing realities can have a very real impact on their lives — and the lives of those around them.

How can we build a healthier relationship with our physicians? First, we can understand that, just as certain types of people with specific personality traits are drawn to teaching, law, firefighting, or any other highly specialized career, many doctors share similar emotional characteristics. Many are perfectionists who have a hard time listening to others, re-evaluating decisions, or admitting to human frailties. But we also need to be aware that we want and even *need* our doctors to have healthy egos. We want them to attack our treatment with confidence and certainty. We want them to hold themselves to the highest standards of performance, and to work as hard as they must work to diagnose and cure our ills. Don't most of us want our doctors to be perfectionists when it comes to our medical care? I certainly do!

WHAT ARE PATIENTS' ROLES IN THEIR OWN HEALTH CARE?

Whether we blame medical schools for creating Doctor Gods out of otherwise caring and committed students, or we blame a medical reimbursement system that drives doctors to see so many patients that ten-minute consultations are the norm, or we blame the doctors themselves for relating to patients with arrogance and assumptions rather than empathy, the problem remains the same. We receive too little time and attention from our caregivers. As we grow more distant, any possibility for a true doctor–patient partnership evaporates. Without that, we are severely limited in our ability to work effectively together. We patients are unhappy, doctors are unhappy, health care suffers, and the costs continue to rise.

In his book *Social Intelligence: The New Science of Human Relationships*, best-selling author Daniel Goleman takes a close look at the importance of the doctor–patient dynamic and its repercussions for both parties. Noting that "humanity too often gets lost in the impersonal machinery of modern medicine," Goleman observes that, given "the relentless fragmentation of medical care, in which patients are shuttled from specialist to specialist," patients often become "the single person in charge of overseeing their medical care, whether they are equipped to do so or not." As Goleman points out, we patients need more from our doctors than just medical expertise and access to cutting-edge medical technology; we also need the compassion and caring that one human being can extend to another — even when we are forced to manage our health care with an ever-changing series of physician specialists and subspecialists.

Strong, healthy doctor–patient collaborations are better for doctors, too. Many doctors say that a desire to help and connect with people was the primary reason they entered medicine in the first place, and some of today's most well-respected medical educators stress that physicians benefit from a closer, more humane approach to medicine. As more newly trained physicians enter the workforce, will the recent emphasis on patient-centered care help heal the damaged doctor–patient relationship? Will growing dissatisfaction with medical errors result in institutional changes to promote a strong relationship between doctors and those they serve? The answers to these questions will tell us much about the issue of nature-versus-nurture in the development of medical narcissism — and about how committed we are as a society to improving our partnerships with our caregivers.

The very idea of working with our doctors as informed partners in health care might seem far-fetched at first glance. We might never have had — or felt that we needed — that kind of relationship with our caregivers in the past. Or it might not seem relevant to our situation. After all, most of us aren't in a Consumer Driven Health Care (CDHC) insurance plan right now, and — given the option — we might never join one. Besides a hefty insurance plan, some of us have great relationships with excellent doctors and put complete trust in their skills and their concern for our welfare. So, really, do we all need to worry about making the effort to become some sort of medical "super consumer"?

The answer to that question is "yes." No matter what kind of health-insurance program, physician, or doctor–patient relationship we enjoy right now, we have no way of knowing what tomorrow may bring. Our insurance company could dump us, our doctor could retire, our employer could transfer us to a new state, or our health needs could change dramatically, and we would be forced to find a new health-care "team." The only player we can depend on forever remaining in our health-care team is us, so we'd better do our best to be a strong and dependable force in that realm.

For many, the wheels of change are already in motion when it comes to personal health care. No more Doctor God (who might more accurately have been called "Mister Fix-it") running the show while we sit back passively and wait for the meds to kick in. No more stumbling obediently from test to test, specialist to specialist, all the while railing against our doctors for not taking the time to understand our symptoms, our needs, and our humanity, and for getting richer as health care becomes less affordable. We don't have the luxury of wallowing in our indignation any longer. Today, many of us have taken on some of the responsibility for remedying both our individual and our national health-care woes.

At its core, America is a self-help nation, and the information age offers the perfect setting for us to put that trait to good use in the pursuit of optimum health. Never in history has the average person in this country had more access to information about diet, exercise, illness, disease, medical treatments, pharmaceuticals, and developing technologies. Not only do we spend time searching for and using printed, broadcast, or online guidelines for diet, exercise, and specific condition-related treatments, we're discussing these ideas with our doctors. If suffering from symptoms, we can jump online and do a quick search to turn up possible causes and, sometimes, basic steps to eliminate the problem. When we need to see a doctor, many of us show up at our appointment with printouts or clippings in hand, ready to weigh our options. The way our doctors respond to this type of active collaboration can tell us a lot about how successfully we can work with them on the day-to-day business of our health.

Patients also are doing more home-based testing and health maintenance tasks than ever before. When we talk about taking care of our health at home, we aren't just referring to the old stand-bys, such as using over-the-counter remedies or adding a treadmill to the family room. Many Americans today are following specific diets aimed at managing such health conditions as high blood pressure, heart disease, hypoglycemia, and macular degeneration. Hundreds of thousands of us routinely check our blood pressure or blood sugar levels, using equipment once considered appropriate only for trained health care professionals.

Ho-hum, you might be yawning, there's nothing new or revolutionary about those diabetes test strips or blood-pressure cuffs. But we can choose from a huge array of home testing and monitoring devices to help track and control the progress of health conditions such as kidney disease, HIV, asthma, and allergies. Monitoring de-vices built into blood pressure cuffs and bathroom scales can transmit results to clinical specialists and disease-management services to help catch developing problems before they become dangerous. Some of these systems include the capability for video and audio conferences with a doctor or clinician. Patients and doctors are collaborating in totally new ways, thanks to the radical changes brought to us by emerging technologies.

Some patients fume when their doctors spend the precious minutes of an office visit typing notes into a computer. Well, whether or not we welcome them, the information about our physical exams those doctors are tapping out is part of a system that promises to revolutionize the business of medicine in America. Many health-care agencies, insurance companies, and employers are lobbying for the creation of a nationwide network of electronic medical records to help track, manage, and coordinate patient care. This system will help in the business of home health care, too. Most agencies want individuals to have access to personal electronic medical records so they can take a more immediate role in monitoring and managing their health programs.

As discussed in an earlier chapter, many agencies hope that electronic medical records will — by eliminating the confusion of badly scrawled notes and making standardized information readily available to any clinician, pharmacist, or physician — help reduce the hundreds of thousands of medical errors that take place in America each year. Networked medical records will also make it easier to deliver targeted treatment plans to individuals for use at home. In 2006, the Department of Health and Human Services secretary Mike Leavitt announced the development of a new tool for delivering downloadable preventative care recommendations to specific individuals online. The tool, called ePSS (Electronic Preventive Services Selector), researches health data within a wide range of topic areas, and uses specific patient characteristics, including age, sex, behaviors, and individual risk factors, to generate specific recommendations. The software can deliver regular updates and ongoing reminders to users' email accounts (it's available right now, too, from the Agency for Healthcare Research and Quality website at www.ahrq.org).

All of these devices, and many others currently in development, are aimed at helping us maintain good health, which is an important part of any real effort to lower the cost of medical care in this country. Today, as much as 80 percent of health-care spending is related to the costs of treating chronic disease. Given the aging nature of our population, we shouldn't expect chronic diseases to become less prevalent. Using home monitoring technology and public education, however, we can expect to dramatically lower the costs of managing these diseases.

Don't think that we're about to turn our doctors out to pasture, though. Any home health-care tool or technology is only as sound as the doctor–patient relationship that backs it up. We'll always need to coordinate our treatment plan with a trained physician or clinician, and nothing will ever replace the professional judgment, evaluation, and treatment of a trained doctor. No computer keyboard or online information bank can take the place of the one-on-one partnerships we forge with our health-care workers, but the better informed we are about our health, the more actively we are engaged in tracking and managing it, the more valuable we can make the time we spend with our doctors. As we grow savvier we'll be in a much better position to know when we need a doctor's intervention, and be better able to work with our doctors in recording, tracking, and controlling problems.

CDHC — CONSUMER MEDICINE BECOMES A MOVEMENT

In any formal discussion about health care today, you're likely to hear patients referred to as "medical consumers." Our country is undergoing a radical change in the way we, as a society, view medicine and the rights, privileges, and responsibilities that go along with its access. From researching our symptoms to maintaining our own medical records, monitoring our vital signs at home, performing routine self-tests, or joining a consumer-driven health-care (CDHC) plan, Americans are taking over more control of their health-care processes and management.

The medical consumer movement has already triggered a dramatic shift in the way we work with our doctors. The popular media knows that Americans are more interested than ever in topics of health and medicine. Magazines, newspapers, and television reports bring up-to-the-minute coverage of developments in medicine to the general public, meaning that sometimes we know about a new test, warning sign, or treatment before our doctor uncovers it in his or her desktop stack of medical journals.

Nor are we as dependent upon our doctors' referrals as we once were. Today, we can go online to search for facilities and specialists offering a variety of potential approaches, amenities, or pricing for treating our medical conditions. And, as many of us are deserted or driven away by traditional insurance programs, we find that we have much greater responsibility in determining which treatment options we will — or can afford to — pursue. In other words, the days of the passive patient are drawing to a close.

At the same time, our nation struggles to cope with the negative effects of medical consumerism. When patients choose to go to a specialty clinic for heart surgeries and other high end procedures, what is the financial impact on general hospitals? How will we regulate the quality and accuracy of medical information that appears online, and how do we know whose opinions to trust? Perhaps most important, how will we work to make sure that we bring the benefits of medical consumerism to the widest sector of our population, so that we don't leave behind the most vulnerable of America's people in a cast-off medical system that no longer has the funding or expertise to care for them? We can't ignore these questions, and we can't afford to "let the chips fall where they may." The way we respond to these issues can teach us a great deal about ourselves, our doctors, and our national attitude toward the business of medicine in America.

Some of the innovations of the medical consumer movement may be short-lived, and others will become the standard for health care in decades to come. Think of this moment in the evolution of medicine as the time when we had to grow up to become full-fledged, responsible adults in caring for our personal health and well-being. We've survived learning the truth about Santa Claus, the Tooth Fairy, and now, Doctor God: good things don't magically appear under a tree or pillow. And no one will look out for us while we sleepwalk through life. Making decisions about health care can be tough, but it's empowering, too.

Create Your Own Health Program

CDHC is the new mantra for many who would like to check the out-of-control rise in medical costs but don't want to go the route of national health-care service in this country. The CDHC movement is fueled by three factors: physicians and patients alike seem to despise HMOs, once seen as the magic bullet for reducing health-care costs; increasing numbers of employers are refusing to foot the bill for spiraling health insurance premiums; and the Internet and direct-to-consumer advertising for drugs and health services are combining to create a class of medical consumers never before seen in this country. The United States may not go the path of CDHC, but many employers are considering this type of plan; some have already made the switch.

These plans come in a variety of forms, but most involve three basic layers of funding and payment. Most CDHC plans include a tax-exempt account (a health service account, or HSA) funded by a set employer contribution and/or enrollee contributions. These accounts are relatively flexible, giving participants a lot of leeway in determining how to use them for medical services. Most of these plans also include a high-deductible insurance feature that will pay for medical services after the deductible is fulfilled.

But between these two payment levels, participants fall into the "donut hole" we've heard so much about in regard to the hotly debated "Part D" Prescription Drug plan added to Medicare in 2005. In a CDHC plan, participants have a period of no benefit coverage that occurs after the account funds have been used and before the participant has paid the out-of-pocket deductible, which typically, is high. Internet support is usually an important part of these plans, allowing participants to get online recommendations and advice when making decisions about purchasing health-care services.

The pros and cons of CDHC are hotly debated, and many (though not all) of the arguments have been tested through the experiences we've had with Part D. Most of the arguments cluster around four main issues: How will CDHC plans affect other health-care plans? Do we really want Americans comparison shopping when choosing health care? Should physicians and medical services be encouraged to compete on costs? Finally, will most Americans actually be capable of participating in such plans?

Many health-care analysts worry that CDHC plans will be the death of the ones that work best for people in most need of health-care funding. Self-funded plans offer the most appeal for younger, healthier, and/or wealthier participants who expect that they can protect themselves against some unusual and catastrophic health problem, while at the same time, pay more of the expenses for routine care, thereby keeping overall health-care insurance investment low.

That reasoning makes sense. Young, healthy people don't have as many health-related expenses as do older or sicker individuals, so why should they pay high premiums for benefits they just don't use as often? But insurance works on the principle of pooled resources. Everyone kicks in a certain premium amount, and some of those people get a lot of benefits from the plan, while others get relatively few. The insurance company, therefore, balances its risks.

But if all of the young and healthy people opt out of any benefit plan, there goes the mix of high- and low-risk participants. As a result, the insurance company no longer has a balanced risk — unless, of course, it removes some of that risk by charging the remaining participants sky-high premiums. In that scenario, older and chronically ill people who are least able to pay those high premiums will be stranded without affordable health care coverage. And that is one of the strongest arguments against CDHC plans.

On the other hand, many employers are refusing to provide any insurance at all now, due to the high cost of premiums in general. A CDHC plan might be the only option for some employees. Plus, the flexibility of an HSA will give all participants more choice in health care than does the traditional HMO, so chronically ill patients might receive better care under a CDHC-type plan.

At the same time, greater consumer involvement typically results in greater consumer oversight. As CDHC plan participants become more directly involved in paying for their health care, you can bet that they'll pay more attention to the types of treatments and services they're using. Unnecessary testing, procedures, and drug therapies won't last long under the intense glare of increased patient scrutiny, and doctors will be forced to learn and explain options and decisions more carefully to a paying "customer."

But is it a good idea for the public to take a bargain-hunter's approach to obtaining health care? We've seen some of the results of the dash for discounts in the retail world. Those mega-marts certainly do offer us low prices, along with a wide cross-section of goods all under one roof. We are a mass-consumer nation and we've learned that if we're willing to sacrifice a bit in quality and convenience, we can drive down prices to rock-bottom levels. Along the way, we've also changed the whole process of merchandising in the United States. In a health-care system shaped by price-conscious consumers, where will the cheapest route take us?

A lot of time and energy in consumer education will have to be invested in consumer education. Shopping for medical services requires an entirely different level of expertise than that used when choosing a new car or microwave. Certainly, we can't let the price of a physician's office visit or a given facility's surgical procedure determine whether or not it's the right one for our medical needs. We must be well versed in our options, possess a good understanding of the potential outcomes of those options, and be ready to dig deep to unearth the facts about our health conditions and the providers, facilities, and treatment plans available to us. In other words, medical consumerism can be a lot of work, and not everyone will be able to do it well.

On the other hand, becoming more involved and knowledgeable about how to take good care of ourselves is effort well spent. The urge to drive down the costs of health care could extend benefits far beyond controlling the price of an office visit or X-ray. One of the best ways to cut those costs is to take good care of ourselves; that means not only eating right and exercising more, but also keeping a watchful eye on our food supply and improving the quality of our natural environment. A CDHC plan might help put an end to the complacent view too many Americans have of health maintenance that says, "What the heck, if it's broken, someone else can pay to fix it." When we're fronting the costs of our lifestyle decisions, maybe we'll be more apt to make good ones.

In the world of economics — and economics has become the driving aspect of health care in America — consumerism translates into competition in the marketplace. That kind of competition can take many forms, but the most common of these is the "price war." At first glance, we might think it would be great if our physicians and hospitals were competing to offer us the best price for an office visit or appendectomy. But is it really wise to encourage our health-care service providers to compete with lower prices, which in many cases will result in lower quality and reduced services?

Traditionally, physicians have been guided by a sense of professionalism and a commitment to quality care. If we define medical services as a consumer "product," some argue, we might very well be giving our medical service providers the green light to cut corners on low-priced services. Yet, others argue that CDHC plans might encourage providers to compete on quality, rather than price. We've seen the risks of a system governed solely by peer review and oversight; when consumers are making choices based on informed comparisons, doctors and the hospitals and clinics they work for might be forced to compete to be the best, rather than the cheapest.

All of these issues make it clear that the success of consumer-driven health care depends on our ability to become savvy medical consumers — *before* disaster strikes. When people are sick, they aren't in the best position to do a lot of shopping around for a good, affordable doctor or medical procedure. In any case, right now, patients can't really comparison shop for a good deal on an MRI. Even if we could access the necessary information on costs, the prices charged for most medical services are pretty well determined by what the insurance companies will pay.

Of course, we can expect that as the medical consumerism movement grows, physicians and medical institutions will become more forthcoming with information about costs, and individual insurance providers will have less sway over the marketplace. But how will that information be made available to us, and will the majority of Americans be able to understand it well enough to do true comparisons of quality and value?

Today, not everyone in America has access to the Internet or the technical ability to use it. While the number of such people is decreasing all the time, it's unlikely that we'll reach a stage anytime soon in which all Americans have the ability to use technology to access information about health care options or to understand the information made available to them. CDHC plans could potentially be even *more* complicated than either HMOs or Medicare's Part D prescription drug plan — and almost all of us have heard the complaints about the complexity of those insurance plans. Many of America's elderly, the poor, those who suffer with severe and/or chronic illnesses, and those who, for whatever reason, simply have poor health literacy might be left out in the cold by the CDHC system.

Still, we know that people can adapt to new ideas and technology. And our nation is unlikely to leave at the curb those who can't fend for themselves in a consumer-driven system. Most of us will take charge of weighing the costs and benefits of the procedures we purchase, while others — individuals and agencies — will assist those who need help in making health-care choices. Evidence points to the many benefits of becoming more engaged in the decisions that govern our lives, thus why we should do so. Otherwise, we've resigned the management of our health to impersonal institutions such as insurance companies or HMO management organizations.

CHAPTER 9
KNOW WHAT'S HAPPENING
IN THE MEDICAL WORLD

ONE OF THE FACTORS destroying the trust given to doctors is the increasing incidence of misdiagnoses and mistreatment within the medical workplace. Few patients today blindly believe that their doctors are giving them good care, as Americans once did.

I personally experienced the consequences of a misdiagnosis. In my late twenties I began to exhibit symptoms that appeared to be the onset of multiple sclerosis. After a battery of tests, the doctors determined I did not have MS, although what caused my symptoms remained a mystery. In time, I recovered, but a few years later had a recurrence. More tests, more "we don't know." One hot-shot physician decided my condition needed a "label" and tagged it as MS, despite earlier proof stating otherwise. He did not discuss it with me; I learned about it later when it was revealed by another doctor. Needless to say, that misdiagnosis created a great deal of consternation and inconvenience in getting it expunged from my medical records and squaring with insurance companies that I did not have this false "pre-existing condition." (After episodes that occurred off and on for a period of about thirty years it was discovered that my problems were caused by an inability to absorb and metabolize Vitamin B.)

MEDICAL MALPRACTICE AND ERRORS

The rise of HMOs resulted in a surge of malpractice suits — many clients in those systems suffered from delayed or denied treatment, and many HMO doctors simply don't have the time to accurately diagnose and treat patients who *do* get in to see them. Even outside the system, the increasing power of the health-care insurance industry to dictate what kinds of treatments and diagnoses will be reimbursed (and at what amounts) has placed a third-party governor squarely at the center of what should be the doctor–patient relationship. And the escalating instances of medical error make us more leery of our clinical caretakers than someone trying to sell us a used car.

This sad scenario helps foster impersonalized attention to patient care, and sets in motion a merry-go-round of bad experiences: medical mistakes spawn malpractice suits; doctors practice defensive medicine to protect themselves from such suits; medical decisions and treatment plans are influenced by the potential for reimbursement and litigation, rather than by individual patient needs and issues; more mistakes are made — and round and round we go.

We find ourselves living in a world where, in any discussion of medical experiences, it's not uncommon to hear at least one person say "I *hate* doctors."

In the introduction to his book *How Doctors Think*, Jerome Groopman notes that during his training he learned from a valued clinician that physicians who want to be excellent in their work must "admit our mistakes to ourselves, then analyze them, and keep them accessible at all times." In the past, however, doctors and medical facilities have been reluctant to admit to errors, let alone create systems for uncovering, analyzing, and avoiding repeating them. Under the glare of an increasingly intense public spotlight, however, denial of the problem of medical errors is no longer an option. We live in an age of avoidance, rather than accountability, where "mistakes were made" substitutes for "I was wrong." These sidesteps succeed more easily in the political arena, however, than they do in the much more intimate setting of a doctor's office. Doctors are learning the lesson most of us learned when we were children: When you make a mistake, you must say you're sorry.

Like members of a twelve-step program, the medical industry realized that its first step toward "healing" was to admit that it has a problem. An important part of that process was to change the way medical institutions respond to patient safety errors. Rather than focusing on denial and damage control, more of those facilities are concentrating on helping patients and their families recover from the effects of medical mistakes.

Writing for *Newsweek* magazine, Lucian Leape, Adjunct Professor of Health Policy at the Harvard School of Public Health, listed the three things he believes victims of medical errors want:

- Disclosure that an error has been made.
- A sincere apology.
- An explanation of what went wrong and what has been done to prevent future incidents.

"Too often," writes Leape, "none of this happens." He cites a survey in which thousands of physicians were presented with sample scenarios involving very serious and definite incidents of medical errors. Less than half of those surveyed said that they would tell a patient that an error had taken place. "Admitting an error exposes a chink in that MD armor," Leape noted.

Leape believes the threat of medical malpractice exacerbates this problem, with lawyers strenuously advising doctors and nurses to remain quiet about errors and to never confess responsibility for mistakes. Conversely, insurers are finding that admitting to mistakes, apologizing for them, and quickly offering victims financial compensation can significantly reduce the number and severity of malpractice suits.

"Doctors have always known it was the right thing to do," Leape concludes. "Now, it appears it's also the smart thing to do." When doctors level with their patients, they build a bridge toward a more effective working relationship. We patients know that anyone can stumble now and then. We're much more forgiving when doctors admit that they know it, too.

Occurrences of medical errors provide some of the strongest evidence of breakdowns in the relationships between doctors and patients. We have no way of knowing precisely how widespread the problem of these errors has become in this country, because many go undetected or unreported, but we know that it is severe. In 2004, Health Grades, Inc., an independent health-care ratings company, reported that nearly 1 million "patient safety issues" occurred during the years 2000 through 2002, and that in-hospital preventable medical errors resulted in nearly 324,000 deaths during that time.

One such incident involved the death of a little girl named Josie King. In January of 2001, the eighteen-month-old girl died at Baltimore's famed Johns Hopkins Children's Center of dehydration and after an injection of methadone — given in spite of a physician's written order to withhold narcotics. How could a little girl die of thirst in one of our nation's most respected children's hospitals under the care of some of our nation's best physicians? In a speech delivered to the Institute for Healthcare Improvement (IHI), Josie's mother, Sorrel King, specifically noted that her daughter's death was the result of "careless human errors," including a breakdown in communication between doctors, nurses, and different medical teams, as well as their refusal to pay attention to the child's condition and her, the mother's, concerns. King held no single person accountable for what she described as "a combination of many errors, all of which were avoidable."

As in the King case, many medical errors result from institutional complexity. As Donald Berwick, MD, president of IHI, stated, "As the machine gets more complicated, there are more ways it can break." Nevertheless, as the "managing member" of a patient's medical team, doctors carry the responsibility for mistakes that occur on their watch. And many errors *are* attributable to physician oversight — particularly those that occur in the doctor's office, rather than in a hospital setting.

A recent report published by the *Annals of Internal Medicine* focused on medical errors that occur in doctors' offices. In that study, researchers found evidence of such errors in more than half of the outpatient cases reviewed, many of which occurred because doctors failed to perform a proper diagnostic test. Further, they didn't follow up on test results, they failed to gather adequate information from the patient, or their physical examination procedure was inadequate.

According to Jerome Groopman, nearly 80 percent of medical mistakes stem from "thinking errors" on the part of doctors and health-care workers, rather than technical failures such as mislabeled X-rays, badly written notes, or false test results.

Patients bear some of the responsibility for errors as well, by failing to provide doctors with complete information about their condition or by failing to keep appointments. And sometimes we patients lie, prompting many doctors to use a multiplier to "correct" the information we supply. As one doctor told us, "If a patient tells me he has one drink a day, I assume he has two or three; if he says he exercises about three times a week, I assume it's once or twice at the most." When the doctor–patient partnership falters on such basic levels, the door to medical errors is left wide open.

IS THAT THE RIGHT DIAGNOSIS?

In America, when mistakes occur, lawsuits soon follow. The costs of malpractice litigation are just one of the negative side-effects of our growing epidemic of medical errors. But how much do we know about its *real* costs?

Many doctors are quick to damn litigation as a terrible tool for managing doctor performance, and let us be the first to agree that its limitations are many. Malpractice suits can be used to punish doctors for problems related to an inevitable bad outcome or understandable human error, rather than negligence. Fears of malpractice claims encourage some doctors and institutions to order unnecessary tests and procedures, a costly practice that we've mentioned called "defensive medicine." Insurers have hiked the price of malpractice insurance so high that some doctors have chosen to leave their practices rather than submit to the costs. Finally, malpractice litigation works to control physician behavior only *after* a tragic error occurs. We can't rely on courts to separate the good doctors from the bad, and the threat of malpractice suits alone isn't enough to protect us from truly sloppy, unprofessional health care.

In spite of its limitations, however, malpractice litigation definitely plays an essential role in uncovering and prosecuting poor physician practices. The medical profession itself promotes peer review as the most effective means of regulation, but without action from patients, other physicians won't necessarily know when a doctor has doled out negligent treatment. Peer-review boards often wait to investigate doctor performance only *after* that doctor is named in a series of malpractice suits. And sometimes, doctors deserve to be punished. When they make careless mistakes that have life-altering results, physicians should pay the professional, personal, and financial consequences.

As any doctor will tell you, insurance premiums — not outlandish court-ordered awards — are the source of much of the cost associated with malpractice. Some reports suggest that insurance companies are both the cause and the beneficiary of skyrocketing premiums. A CBS news story looked at the case of one physician whose malpractice premiums climbed from $23,000 in 2002 to $47,000 in 2003, and had been quoted at $84,000 for 2004. The insurance industry places the blame for these rates on the legal system and (get ready for the cliché) "skyrocketing malpractice awards."

But the CBS report found that some experts believe the insurance industry artificially inflated malpractice premium prices in an effort to recover its investment losses during that period. It pointed out that when OB-GYN malpractice premiums doubled from 2001 to 2002, payouts to victims of malpractice were, in fact, declining. At the same time, insurance companies were losing large amounts of money on their investments (a major source of their income). Although many have claimed that "junk and frivolous lawsuits" are major cost drivers in the delivery of health care in this country, little hard data backs up that claim. After President George W. Bush stated that malpractice award caps could save the Department of Health and Human Services over $100 billion annually, the General Accounting Office (GAO) and Congressional Budget Office (CBO) did their own analysis; the CBO found "no evidence that restrictions on tort liability reduce medical spending."

What about the related, very real costs of defensive medicine? As

Sick of Doctors?

Time magazine's Nancy Gibbs and Amanda Bower note, our medical system suffers from "a dangerous impulse toward excess" as doctors over-test patients — once again, relying on technology over human contact to diagnose medical conditions. Is this tendency toward over-testing prompted solely by fears of malpractice? Or do doctors rush to testing because it's the more lucrative approach? Remember, taking an hour to talk through symptoms with a patient will pay a doctor only the cost of a routine office visit; spending ten minutes with that patient, then assigning a series of tests, can be much more profitable. Doctors can use defensive medicine to protect income, therefore, as well as for protection against charges of malpractice.

Ultimately, perhaps one of the main victims of malpractice litigation is the doctor–patient relationship. Whether we are consciously aware of it or not, the potential for malpractice claims hovers over our interactions with caregivers. And many doctors cite the demands of meeting the rising costs of malpractice insurance and fear of such litigation as a factor in burnout and decisions to take early retirement.

Patient Safety Is Not an Option

Americans from all walks of life are scrambling to find solutions to the lingering problems of medical errors. But no system can prevent people — and that includes doctors and other medical personnel — from making mistakes. Instead, we have to focus on creating processes that will catch those errors before they can result in harm.

Hospitals and medical centers around the country are realizing that rather than relying on the infallibility of individuals providing health care, they need to institutionalize the processes of patient safety. The Josie King Patient Safety Program at Johns Hopkins and the Condition H program at Shadyside Hospital in Pittsburgh are just two examples of systems designed to engage medical staff at all levels, along with patients and their families, in the effort to monitor and safeguard the treatment of in-patient clients.

Johns Hopkins apologized to the Kings for their daughter's unnecessary death, an act of contrition that many institutions historically have resisted. But the King family wanted more than a *mea culpa*. They used part of the settlement money received from Hopkins to fund the hospital's Josie King Patient Safety Program — a program that has installed multiple teams throughout the Children's Center that work to predict and avoid patient risks. These teams focus strictly on safety, and they share their experiences and findings with each other to make sure that everyone in the medical center is aware of the potential for human and system errors in all parts of the treatment areas. Shadyside Hospital's Josie King Condition H program enables family members who become concerned about a dramatic change in a patient's condition to trigger a call that will bring a rapid response team to the patient's aid. *Newsweek*'s Claudia Kalb quotes Sorrel King as saying, "The bottom line is that [the programs] would have saved Josie."

Such approaches are one way to make the prevention of medical errors everyone's privilege and responsibility. They encourage doctors to work more closely with patients, families, nurses, and other medical personnel in monitoring and tracking patient treatment and progress. Most important, they encourage everyone in the medical workplace to ask questions and raise concerns without fear of angering the attending physician.

One thing is certain: If you think doctor dissatisfaction is *their* problem, not ours, you're wrong. Early retirement of physicians, avoidance of unpopular subspecialties, and burnout are the very real prices we patients pay.

When physicians become unhappy with their workplace, many are tempted to retire early or leave medicine entirely in pursuit of a different career. In July of 2000, Jennifer Proctor studied the impact of job dissatisfaction on doctors and on America's medical services industry. She found that nearly half of doctors age fifty or older were planning to leave medicine by 2004, and 53 percent had closed their practices to new patients. When doctors decide that it's easier to just cash out and leave their field, they take with them their years of experience and training. The more often that happens, the wider grows the hole in the fabric of our nation's health care.

Intense dissatisfaction within an area of specialization can discourage medical students from pursuing it and result in shortages in that field. In the 1990s, for example, surveys revealed growing career dissatisfaction among anesthesiologists. By 2001, professional journals were reporting a shortage there, even though anesthesiology remained one of the more lucrative areas of medicine. Few of us want to see shortages develop in any sector of medicine, particularly within the surgical subspecialties and emergency medical fields reporting high levels of discontent today. Nevertheless, that evidently is exactly what is happening.

If we face an exodus of experienced, highly qualified physicians, we're left to seek health care from those who remain — and many experts express concern that if current trends continue, the quality of that remainder might steadily deteriorate. That's troubling, considering that this country is facing an unprecedented spike in health care demand, as its crowded baby boomer population forges ahead into old age.

While some physicians abandon their profession to escape the pressures of a deteriorating work environment and others find ways to maintain or even improve their working conditions, a significant number of them today simply struggle on in dissatisfaction. These physicians are ripe for burnout, a condition that involves emotional exhaustion and isolation, a lack of concern for others in the workplace (both patients and colleagues), and a cynical and detached attitude toward the field of medicine itself. Doctor burnout can contribute to depression, anxiety, impaired memory and performance, drug abuse, and even suicide. Unfortunately, today's medical workplace is primed with problems that fuel this fire.

Consider, for example, the movement in many large medical organizations toward turning over routine procedures and patient care to nurse practitioners and medical assistants, leaving only the more serious problems and patient issues for the doctors' attention.

While that arrangement makes good financial sense, it also means that doctors are going to face higher concentrations of more difficult health problems. They also will have fewer successes, and that fact alone can make doctors' work more challenging, less satisfying, and more stressful.

As noted earlier, studies show that many physicians are perfectionists and want a high level of control in their work. Those who possess those traits find it difficult to cope with very common issues in the medical workplace today. The resulting stresses can seriously cripple a doctor's performance and lead to burnout. Burnt-out doctors can't take care of their patients or themselves — and that's not a good prescription for anyone.

GMP — GOOD MEDICAL PRACTICE

The medical industry and its associated organizations are fully aware of the need for better accountability in physician practice and patient care. In March of 2005, the Federation of State Medical Boards convened a summit of leaders from a variety of health-care-related fields to discuss the future of physician accountability and self-regulation. Over the next two years, the alliance expanded its participants to include medical schools and institutions, patient advocacy groups, consumer unions, insurers, medical suppliers, law schools, and a wide variety of other groups with interests and investments in this critical issue. During that time, through a series of surveys and studies, the alliance compiled a document known as *Good Medical Practice — USA*, or, simply, GMP, modeled after Great Britain's General Medical Council *Good Medical Practice* document of 2006. In September 2007, the alliance released a draft of the document to doctors and other stakeholders in America's medical community so they could begin to use and provide feedback on its guidelines. (As of July of 2008, a full version of the GMP became available for viewing and comment online at www.gmpusa.org; registration is required, but it is free of charge.)

The GMP draft's guidelines cover a range of important issues that shape the quality of physician care and the doctor–patient collaboration. In the draft's opening, the alliance members state that "We, members of the medical profession, believe that every patient is entitled to a good doctor, one who possesses the essential skills and knowledge, and who demonstrates the behaviors that serve patients and society as a whole." The document's chapters include guidance for six basic competencies: Patient Care, Medical Knowledge and Skills, Practice-based Learning and Improvement, Interpersonal and Communication Skills, Professional Behavior, and Systems-based Practice. The final GMP document will outline the basic expectations of the medical community and its regulators for all doctors practicing medicine in the United States. Doctors who deviate from the guidelines will be expected to "explain and justify" their actions. The alliance urges all medical educators and regulators to incorporate the guidelines into their missions, but it also urges the public to hold those agencies and members of the medical profession to the principles and standards it sets forth.

Although physicians and non-physicians alike participated in the alliance, the draft GMP is careful to separate the guidelines developed by lay people from those developed by medical professionals. The two-page segment that outlines "Patient's Perspective" on expectations for physician competence and behavior is not listed as one of the document's six chapters, which contain what are described as "physician-developed principles." In other words, while the GMP is an important step forward in calling doctors to increased accountability and more structured self-regulation, it still reflects the medical profession's unwillingness to submit to regulations put forward by anyone outside their ranks. Nevertheless, the GMP represents a valuable tool for patients and members of the medical industry alike.

The Patient's Perspective section states among other things that we expect our doctors to:

- Have effective and up-to-date clinical skills and to communicate and collaborate with other physicians and practitioners on issues affecting our care.

- Treat us with dignity, civility, and respect.
- Listen attentively and actively to our concerns.
- Be empathetic and responsive to our fears and provide emotional support.
- Explain things to us in understandable terminology.
- Provide clear and prompt answers to our questions.
- Involve us in decisions about tests, treatments, and other care options.
- Respond promptly to our calls.
- Disclose conflicts of interest and commercial relationships or any other factor that might impact medical advice and treatment plans.

If these guidelines sound too good to be true, remember that they're only a small portion of the document's complete outline of expectations. Further guidelines describe principles for working with colleagues, providing compassionate patient care, gathering complete information about patient histories, preserving personal (the physician's) health and stability, maintaining skills and understanding limitations, and improving patient-care practices. Important standards are given for continuing education and skill enhancement — crucial standards, given that some fourteen states fail to require physicians to participate in continuing medical education. Far from allowing doctors to blame "the system" for failures in health care, the GMP sets forth a series of principles aimed at making doctors accountable for learning the structure of the health-care systems in which they work and finding ways to effectively call on those system resources to provide the best possible patient care.

No one realistically expects the GMP document to solve all of the ills involving physician competence or the doctor–patient relationship. Given that these guidelines will require physicians to control their egos and invest more time in the human aspects of patient care, we can safely assume that the GMP will generate controversy in the medical community. When the draft document was first released, an article in the *AAMC* [Association of American Medical Colleges] *Reporter* quoted Jordan J. Cohen, MD, former AAMC president and a participant in the alliance, as saying, "I wouldn't be surprised if the document raised some questions. The degree to which the profession can address all these issues is uncertain."

Regardless, the document's creators are hopeful that the GMP will become a guiding force within the culture of medicine, and that doctors and patients both will benefit from its influence. AAMC vice president and alliance participant Carol Aschenbrener, MD, has described the GMP as a "modern-day explication for the Hippocratic oath," and stressed that it is intended to be "embraced by the medical profession, not imposed."

CHAPTER 10
REJOICE WHEN YOU
FIND A WINNER!

WE ALL KNOW THAT the only way to gain a clear and objective view of a story is to hear all sides.

I have had the great fortune to know two outstanding physicians. One, Howard Harris, was Medical Director of the Neonatal Intensive Care Unit at Methodist Hospital in Indianapolis, and an Associate Clinical Professor of Pediatrics at IU School of Medicine. The other is Timothy Kelly, an otolaryngological surgeon with one of the largest ear, nose, and throat group practices in the state of Indiana; he also is a Clinical Professor at the Indiana University Medical Center. Despite being all too aware of the issues facing the medical profession today, both gentlemen are among the majority of physicians who say they are happy with their career choice. The doctors graciously agreed to let me interview them in 2008.

Harris and Kelly chose quite different professional paths, but they share a deep and unshakable commitment to their patients and the practice of medicine.

THERE ARE GOOD DOCTORS! MEET TWO OF THEM

Howard Harris, MD

Howard Harris began his career in medicine in 1968, when he entered his internship at the Philadelphia Children's Hospital. At the time of our interview, he was part of a group practice of five physicians; Harris was an independent member of Clarian Health Partners, while his four colleagues were employed by Riley Hospital and IUSM. (Harris has since retired.)

159

"I used to, in the past, have patients who were only my patients," Harris said. "Now we have five people in this practice and we rotate, so multiple physicians establish relationships with the patients."

Harris completed his residency at the Philadelphia Children's Hospital in 1971, then — after a stint in the army — completed a fellowship in 1975. He takes care of newborns — tiny "premies" who have a better chance of living now than they would have at any previous time in history. Harris was in the first group of physicians to take the board exams in neonatology.

"Some of the people who wrote the textbooks took the boards with me," he remarked. "Of course, it's changed a lot. We have better ways of feeding the babies, and we have better equipment. These babies get diseases due to deficiencies in their lungs, and we have better ventilators and surfactants that help to give them a better chance of survival. We've learned a lot."

Harris fell in love with neonatology almost from his first clinical experiences. "As an intern, I had some very sick babies; I was thrown into a crazy situation at Pennsylvania Hospital, and I was on my own my first weekend there. But I really liked it. I decided that internal medicine wasn't appealing to me, because the diseases are long-term and don't necessarily improve. With children, though — they can get better, so I felt like I could really make a difference by treating them. I learned early on that if you're not comfortable with emergencies, this work can be overwhelming. In an emergency, someone has to be in charge who is very organized and who can manage the chaos. And I'm a very organized person."

He was the first of his family to receive a formal degree in medicine — but he wasn't the last.

"My grandfather on my mother's side coming from Russia was a lay physician, but he had no formal training. My father was in the furniture business, and my brother sells automobiles. Today, I have one son who is a dermatologist, and another who is a doctor of Chinese medicine."

Studies indicate that some doctors today advise their children not to go into medicine because of rising costs, loss of autonomy, and stagnant incomes, but Harris sees those as problems more relevant to individual personality and career goals, rather than as issues that plague every medical workplace.

"Those are real problems," he noted, "but many specialties — such as surgery — are more affected than mine. Personality tests typically class pediatricians as having altruistic personalities. Of course, in this country, we like to talk about how anything having to do with mothers and babies is so important to us. But if you then look at any program or profession having to do with mothers and babies, you'll find that it's on the lowest end of the pay scale. Pediatricians are the lowest paid of all doctors, but in general, physicians who go into medicine looking for money and power are probably very disappointed.

"The days when medicine clearly could give you a high money return are over. You have to spend a lot of time and money to go into medicine. Today, there's a better chance to make big money going into business or other fields."

Harris let his sons make their own decisions about whether or not to enter the field of medicine. "My son didn't want to go into neonatology," Harris laughed, "because he saw what that was like. He's a dermatologist, and his life certainly is much easier than mine. He has every Monday morning and every Wednesday off. My son has had two or three [after-hours] phone calls in three years, versus my sometimes ten calls per night when I first started.

"Dermatology is the most sought-after residency in medicine — I heard that 48 percent of a recent Yale medical school class wanted to go into dermatology. For the entire nation, there are approximately one thousand dermatology residency places available each year compared to the over twenty-two thousand residencies in internal medicine. By keeping the flow of dermatologists restricted, they determine that these will be highly sought, highly paid positions."

Harris also cited other changes in the practice of medicine that have reshaped the experience of being a doctor.

"Today," he said, "resident physicians have rules about how many hours they can work. Eighty hours used to be a light schedule. When I first started, I worked every other night and every other weekend.

I'm not sure how I got through my marriage because I was tired all the time. When I wasn't at work I wanted to sleep. I used to fall asleep eating dinner — I would sleep anywhere. Physicians don't want to do that anymore.

"Of course," he continued, "there were some benefits to working all of those hours. We saw a lot of patients and could follow through a lot of disease processes. Now, when your allotted time is up, you have to leave, even if you're in the middle of surgery. The Yale surgical residency program was put on probation because they weren't following the rules. The guidelines now limit resident physicians to eighty hours in a week; these limitations are dictated by the residency review programs in each area of specialization. When your program is under review for accreditation, these people come and check, and they're very strict; they make sure you're following these rules. And it applies to all fields — pediatrics, surgery, and so on."

Harris noted that residency work-hour rules have also resulted in more specialist nurses covering jobs previously assigned to residents. That change, in turn, has given team-medicine a boost, something he's not opposed to at all.

"I've always practiced team medicine," he said. "From very early on, I decided that the nurse had to be my friend. I saw some people who didn't have the nurses on their side, and things weren't as good for those people. I work with lots of people every day — respiratory specialists, neonatal nurses, other pediatric specialists. You have to be able to work with people."

Not all of Harris' colleagues share his opinion.

"In the past, doctors made all the decisions — there were never questions about processes or costs. No one said, 'Let's do it another way.' Physicians just did what they wanted; they were captains of the whole thing and nobody questioned it. The people who trained them acted that way, so they acted that way as well. Today, you just can't get by with that behavior. There were doctors at this hospital who cursed and threw things at nurses. No one said anything. Now, lawsuits are brought for that type of behavior.

"Doctors today are taught an entirely different point of view by the people who train them," Harris continued. "They know they have to change. The control of insurance companies over what you bill and how you bill is totally different from how it was in the past. I don't have to worry about that, because I don't have to bill for individual patients [Harris was on salary]. My son the dermatologist does have to bill, though, so he's had to learn how to deal with it. We have a lot of talk about individual cost per patient and whom we work with. The physicians we're training realize that's all part of the process. If asked to make tremendous changes, that's much more difficult than simply learning to operate this way from the beginning."

Harris acknowledged that changes in insurance oversight have affected the delivery of health care.

"The insurance companies will pay for procedures, but not for time to think. You have to see patients very quickly, get them in and out. Many groups or hospitals keep track of productivity based on the number of patients you're seeing in a set time. Some physicians do very well in this system. Cardiologists do very well on the scale, as do surgeons or plastic surgeons who don't have to work with insurance. But it's a terrible system for pediatricians — they have to spend a lot of time talking to families, and consultation time doesn't generate a lot of money. And now Medicare is squeezing tighter and tighter.

"People don't get much time to see the doctor. As a result, some rate nurses better than doctors because they spend more time talking to the nurse. There's a lot of unhappiness among physicians because of this. Physicians in the past — in the 1930s and '40s — were very well-respected but they didn't make fabulous sums of money. Then insurance came along and the money rolled in. At some point, doctors gave away their ability to be in control to insurance companies, but they weren't aware of it because they were doing so well. By the time insurance companies began dictating time and procedures, it was too late; physicians will never get that control back."

Many analysts believe that health care in the United States has become a tiered system, with one level of care for the wealthy and another for the poor and uninsured. Howard Harris understands that viewpoint.

"It's true. People still get care. They can still go to the emergency room to see someone but it's the worst form of health care imaginable. Emergency rooms don't give doctors or patients a chance to do well in the health-care process. For example, you can't handle diabetes, high blood pressure, or heart disease from an emergency room. Without insurance, you can't get preventive care, so all that's left is the emergency room. People are using the ER as their primary doctor because they don't have primary-care physicians.

"On the other hand," he continued, "if people don't pay at all, they don't value the service. One excellent physician's experience reminded me of that. Most of this doctor's patients are on Medicaid. They won't come in for appointments, but they'll call him in the middle of the night about things like rashes. Now, he's hardened to them, and he says, 'Go to the ER.' His whole attitude has changed because his patients don't have any respect for him as a person."

Harris witnessed other changes in medicine over the course of his career, including some evolution in the attitudes of doctors themselves. His other son and his daughter-in-law, Mitchell and Erica Harris, are doctors of Chinese medicine who have established a successful practice in Indianapolis.

"The Midwest lags behind the coasts in acupuncture and Chinese medicine," Harris noted, "but my son Mitchell has gotten to know many physicians in different specialties, so he's aware of what works well with Chinese therapies. He's working with several physicians; in fact, there's an OB at Clarian North who has done some acupuncture and apparently is very busy. Physicians are referring patients to her for acupuncture. It would have been impossible to integrate Chinese and Western medicine twenty-five years ago because of the way doctors were back then. The ego-driven doctor could not collaborate like this. The changes in the culture of medicine make this kind of collaboration possible. There's an opening of minds and experiences on both sides.

While many of the surgeons he worked with were nothing like that old Doctor God stereotype, Harris conceded that some are still out there.

"In my medical class, there was a cardiovascular surgeon who was like that," he said. "One of the students forgot to tape his eyeglasses on, and they dropped down into the operating field. The surgeon threw the glasses to the floor, stepped on them and crushed them. There was a very famous surgeon at Ohio State who decided he didn't like one of the medical students he was teaching. He had the nurse tape the student to an IV pole. That type of behavior was not uncommon in the past. These people were in total control and no one said anything."

Harris was happy to note that those days have passed.

"That kind of attitude isn't accepted anymore. Surgeons are just nicer people now than they were in the past. Everyone is a human being, a person. I'm not a god; I'm just like everyone else who needs that human connection and understanding. I have special training, but other than that, I'm not anything special.

"The down side is that I don't know where I see medicine going, and frankly, I'm a little concerned. There are still some very, very good medical students and residents, but overall, I don't think that medicine attracts the brightest and the best anymore. Many of those people are going into business or law, which pay better money and operate under fewer regulations. Many of the brightest students today want to make money, so they get their degree in four years and begin making money."

Harris always enjoyed his work but acknowledged that as he grew older, it became harder for him, especially if he had to go in at two in the morning, then work the next day, or had an entire week of being on call.

One constant throughout his life, though, was that family was always his number-one priority.

"Family has to be at the top. My wife told me that when she married me, she thought my job would be the most important thing in my life. She was thrilled when she saw that the family was first. It took a lot of work to be there for my family, to go to my sons' games, and so on, but I knew it was important and I did it. It takes a lot of hard work to raise a family, but it's worth it. My family still has wonderful relationships; we love to spend time together, we kiss when we greet each other, and I think it's marvelous. But I think a lot of physicians don't realize how important it is. You work better with everyone when you have strong relationships at home."

Harris went on to talk about the benefits of a health-care system — and a national culture — that places more focus on family health and relationships.

"In Scandinavian countries, both mother and father get six months off with pay after a baby is born; here mothers fight for six weeks. Then we're surprised about what happens with kids — delinquencies and so on. Look at the way kids are treated; mothers and fathers both working, and no one has time for the kids.

"That's the thing that bothers me the most about what we do in neonatology. We spend a lot of time on these babies, and I have real concern about what will happen with them when they leave. The population has changed from when I first started working. Few of the parents I saw then had drug problems. Now, it's not uncommon at all to see mothers who smoke marijuana or do cocaine. Many kids are taken from their parents and put into foster homes. We can take care of them when they're born, but who will take care of these kids after they leave the hospital?"

Timothy Kelly, MD

Timothy Kelly is a self-described "head and neck surgeon" — a member of Otolaryngology Associates, the largest ear, nose, and throat (ENT) group in the state of Indiana. He spoke with us in his offices at Clarian North, Indianapolis' newest and most lavish medical facility.

"We have offices at Community North, on the Westside, downtown, and south — all around," Kelly noted. As a result of working in multiple locations and types of facilities around the city, he sees patients from a variety of socioeconomic groups.

Kelly grew up in Traverse City, Michigan, the sixth of seven children of a dentist.

"I'll be blunt," he said. "Where I grew up, the smart guys and gals went into medicine or law. They didn't go into business. The business people I knew when I was a kid owned a cherry farm, shoe store, restaurant. I did well in high school; I was the valedictorian of my graduating class. I also did well in undergrad at Michigan State; after two years I applied to and was accepted at med school at the University of Michigan, so I started medical school at age twenty.

"At the end of my second year of medical school I was first in my class. The assistant dean of the school called me into his office and asked me what I wanted to be; I told him that I planned to go into family practice and return to Traverse City to practice. He said, 'No, you're not the type of person for that; you need to have a specialty.' That wasn't a slap in the face for family docs; Ann Arbor just had a very different atmosphere at that time — they put out specialists. I thought, 'What will it be?' I'm an impatient man, so I thought I'd become a surgeon. Now, nearly every general surgery resident that I knew at that time either was divorced or in the process of getting a divorce, and that's not my kind of lifestyle. I looked at the other surgical specialties, and decided that ENT offered the best mix of surgery, practice, and a good lifestyle. Also, it's very intricate surgery, and I liked that; there's microscopic stuff, simple stuff, major surgery — it's a good mix.

"In my residency, I did two years of general surgery, then three or four more years of ENT, which I did here at the Indiana University Medical Center. I was going to go back to a fellowship in Ann Arbor because I wanted to teach at the University of Michigan, but my wife became very ill with breast cancer and passed away; that was sixteen years ago. I was approached with an offer I couldn't refuse in Indianapolis — a wonderful group of professionals. I love to teach, but I also love to practice medicine. Here, I get to do both. Fourth-year residents spend their whole year with our group. I'm now in my fifteenth year of practice with this group. Today, I'm remarried, and my wife and I together have five children."

Kelly says that, for him, being a doctor is more than just a career. "It's my life. I'm not a 'mister' anymore. I don't turn it off. I go on vacation and I think about the surgeries that I've done. If something happens, they call me and I take care of it. I don't go home and forget about my work. My neighbor cut his lip, and I sewed it up on the kitchen table!

"I'm a perfectionist," he continued. "There's no kind of halfway at home or work. If I'm relaxing, I'm very relaxed; when at work, I'm on the job. My colleagues know that I am rarely late. When I'm here, I'm seeing patients. I don't stop to chit-chat in the hall; I do my work, then go home. When people come in, they expect service. People who come to see me are busy. They don't want to wait — sometimes even fifteen minutes. I start early, I go-go-go, and I'm out of here — usually at five o'clock.

Necessity taught Kelly the discipline of balancing family and work life early in his career.

"When I started in practice, I was a newly single father of three kids, ages one, two, and six. I told my nurse I don't ever want my practice to get in the way of getting home. I had a nanny, and I had to get her home on time, too. And managing your work hours is a good practice, anyway. I take Wednesday afternoon off and don't come in here unless someone twists my arm and wants me to be here for a special reason. I love my downtime, and I need it.

"My experiences have taught me that life is too short. I used to be a typical type-A personality, driven all the time; then I realized that I have to enjoy my life, too. Come four o'clock on Saturday, if my wife — who is a busy person — is doing something in the house, I tell her come outside and sit on the deck with me and have a cocktail. 'I'm out here and I want some company!' You have to plan for downtime or it won't happen. You can't hang out at the office forever. My goal is to go home and have dinner every night with my family. When I'm at work, I'm regimented."

Many surgeons strive to attain that kind of regimentation, both in their schedules and approach to surgery. As Atul Gawande, a surgical resident at a Boston hospital, noted in his award-winning book, *Complications,* the best surgeons work like finely tuned machines. Kelly agrees. "I like to be mechanized, because the more consistently

I do something, the less likely there will be variance in the outcome. If I find a way that I can do something better, certainly I change. But I've been told that in the OR I am very particular, and I say that's right. In the OR, you don't want anything else.

"The OR is much different than you might expect; we banter a bit, we have music on, and so on. I enjoy myself there. But when it comes to cutting, it's gotta be 'this way' — not 'kinda this way,' but '*this way*.' There are definitely surgeons who abuse their position by lashing out when they're under stress. Nobody makes a better decision when they lose their cool. People know I'm stressed when I become very quiet. I'm focused. I've had to say, 'I need a little quiet,' because the music is going or they're talking about things that have nothing to do with medicine. I'll remind them that this may be routine to us, but it's not routine to this patient."

Kelly said that he rarely encounters doctors who are clearly egotistical, detached, non-empathetic, demanding, or who generally seemed to consider themselves apart from the rest of humanity.

"Most of the physicians I interact with are really nice people. There are certain surgeons who have certain reputations, of course, but ENTs have their own type of personality. At the University of Michigan, we're referred to as the 'gentleman surgeons' because we tend to be just a little more laid back and happy. Partially, I suppose that's because we have good jobs and good lifestyles.

"Cardiovascular surgeons," Kelly added, "are clearly at another end of the spectrum; they really can be tough. They handle people's hearts every day, and I suppose that could make you egocentric sometimes — maybe with reason. Orthopedic surgeons also can be pretty tough.

"Urologists and ENTs and ophthalmologists are about the same. The types of surgery we do sometimes can have life-altering outcomes, especially with appearance. But we deal with a lot of kids, and you can't be rough and tough and egocentric with kids; they won't want to work with you and you'll lose business. And that can re-orient your behavior and attitude quickly because I think economics also plays some role in that Doctor God behavior — I really do."

Still, Kelly was quick to point out that doctors need a high level of self-confidence.

"You have to have a very intact ego to do certain things in medicine. If you're not confident and self-aware, you aren't in the right field. Confidence can go hand-in-hand with ego, but empathy and other such qualities are much more evident in doctors today. I see these qualities in the residents I teach; they have much different personalities than what used to be the norm among residents.

"There are some minuses with these changes, though," Kelly added. "Medical residents today aren't as committed as residents once were, which goes back to the economics of medicine. You used to work your tail off, but you knew you'd do well. There was a saying, 'If you're available, affable, and able, you can just hang out your shingle and you'll do well.' Now there are some good people out there who aren't doing well — they're not busy, and you have to be busy. You can't have a lot of downtime because you have to pay the bills."

Is *paying the bills* harder for doctors now?

"You get less per patient today than you used to," Kelly said. "The average salary or income in our group in 1980 was the same as it is today — and I'm not talking about adjusting dollars for inflation. We make the same salary. That's why, now, most bright, capable people are talking about getting their MBA and going into business. Why not? They can make the same or more than a surgeon, without all of the stress. My niece is a very bright girl; she was pre-med and wanted to go into pediatrics, and her advisor said, 'No, go into dentistry. You'll make more than you will as a pediatrician.'

Isn't it a *good* thing, though, that fewer people are entering the field of medicine solely because they view it as a passport to wealth and power?

"It should be," Kelly admitted, "but you still have to attract people who are bright and determined enough. Going through medical school is rigorous; to get through it, to be committed enough to get all of those years of training, and to emerge with $100K or $200K worth of debt that you'll be repaying for thirty years — you just aren't going to get the best and the brightest choosing to do that.

Rejoice When You Find a Winner!

"Someone told me once that physicians don't go into their field for money, but let's face it, they used to know it was there. You can get yourself through some pretty rough nights and long hours and tough times knowing that you'll emerge into something that will offer a solid life. But now, [as a doctor] you find yourself having to make some hard decisions that you wouldn't normally make. You think, 'Gosh, can I take this case because it's going to take me away from some of my better-paying cases?' I don't want to make those decisions. I just want to make people better. That's what I do — take care of patients."

As a medical educator, Kelly has seen the impact of changes in medical training today.

"The hour restrictions definitely have changed things. You still have to learn the same amount of information, maybe more, but the hours make it easier. And they are teaching, like at IU, relationship-centered care. ENT is a small field in this state, and it's one of the toughest to get into — which is why we're so busy. We do get really good quality people. But even our students realize that there are hour restrictions, only so many weekends a month."

Kelly also discussed the rising numbers of women in medical practice — a movement often referred to as "the feminization of medicine." Some medical industry analysts have speculated that, because women typically are less willing than men to sacrifice their family and private life toward the pursuit of a career, this trend could have a significant impact on the field of medicine in the years to come.

"We have four women in our practice, and in terms of productivity [because of shorter hours], three of those four are the bottom in our group. But we don't care, because they're good physicians and we like them, and we don't see a need to push them.

"The only concern I have," he added, "is that a lot of money goes into training a physician — especially at a public school. If the public spends all of those tax dollars training a physician and that physician practices for just a few years before deciding to drop out, that's probably not good for society. Of course, many men also drop out to take on other careers, so that concern isn't solely related to women in medicine."

Kelly also acknowledged that some doctors have trouble dealing with the shift toward team medicine.

"It can be difficult, depending on their roles," he said. "They say that organizing a group of doctors is like herding cats. You have a bunch of type-A, driven, confident people who all think they're right. Getting them to line up in a row isn't easy. When you're the one heading up the team, it's different; but otherwise. . .

"The situation between doctors and nurses also has changed a lot," Kelly noted. "Most of the younger doctors don't have nurses because it's too expensive, so they have medical assistants instead. There's definitely a difference and that's why I'm willing to pay what I have to for my nurse, Judy. Nurses can take a lot of work off doc-tors — like calling patients for follow-up — that probably isn't necessary for a doctor's level of skill, and that doctors aren't as good at, either. My patients receive better care because of Judy. They may come to see me, but they stay as patients because of both Judy and me.

"Nurses are driven to help people, and I feel for them now. It's especially difficult for floor nurses. Inpatient care is intense these days; it isn't just a gallbladder patient who needs you to give him a sponge bath and fill his water bottle. Inpatient care involves needy patients, and you have four assistants who are trying to run around and attend to everything. Those assistants may not be aware when things go bad, and you have to be responsible for things that can go bad very quickly."

What happens when things go bad in a health-care setting? In a study published by the *New England Journal of Medicine* of a number of New York hospitals regarding doctor error, 1 percent of admissions had problems that were directly related to that.

How do bad physicians get culled out?

"Hopefully," Kelly said, "a 'bad' doctor's reputation gets through to the nurses. We also hope that primary-care physicians become aware of these doctors' bad results. The market will then force them to change. Unfortunately, in an area where there aren't many good physicians practicing within a given medical specialty, that kind of market-force pressure might not happen."

What about problems market forces simply can't address? Doctors are more likely than patients to know when a physician has made an egregious error, and — as the old saying goes — "doctors bury their mistakes." If most patients have no way of knowing if a bad outcome was the result of negligence or substandard care, rather than something that was simply unavoidable, the market may be ineffective in weeding out physicians with repeated problems of poor performance. Can peer review provide the necessary safeguards the market lacks?

"If a bad physician gets sued, that has an impact," Kelly replied. "But if it doesn't produce a lawsuit, other physicians may not be able to help; in fact, they may never know. No one ever knows everything a doctor does in the course of treating a patient, even though they might look at the results and wonder. For example, there's a city here in Indiana where we know that some physicians just aren't good — maybe their judgment isn't good. I see people from there who have had surgery and think, 'What did this surgeon *do*?' But I don't know what I can do about that, unless I run across a really gross error; then I could go to the State Board of Health. At the same time, litigation is a horrible tool for managing doctors and eliminating bad ones. It doesn't equate, because people are not machines. Things happen, and it doesn't mean anything was done horribly or inaccurately.

"I sit on plenty of panels and I have found against the physician where there was obvious evidence that the physician was negligent. But I have to admit that the peer-review process isn't always efficient, probably because many physicians don't want to be confrontational with colleagues. As a doctor, you can't ignore that behavior, because you took the oath. Yet, we've had situations in our group where we've had to take a physician aside and tell him his behavior isn't acceptable. Sometimes we've gone through training as a group — impaired physician classes — to help improve one individual's behavior. We also have a policy, so that maybe as a group we can commit to supporting the improvement of our physicians."

Kelly also noted that patient opinion is important for simply keeping a doctor in business.

"I think most people expect that any doctor trained in the United States is going to do a good job. But referral is largely a matter of word of mouth. If a patient says, 'Dr. So-and-So is a jerk,' it takes only that one time and that doctor might be off the list of referrals. If, however, they say the doctor took good care of them, we remember that, too. Being nice — that's another way that things are changing. You can't be busy if people don't want to work with you."

What is his perception of the direction medical service delivery is going in this nation?

"I have fears," Kelly said, "that some physicians are to the point of giving up. They're tired of dealing with their insurance companies. But then, a single payer would be the government, and that isn't good for anybody. I have fears that we've gotten to the point where perhaps insurers will have some list of physicians that meet their criteria, but we don't know what those criteria are. And that's going to push a lot of good physicians out of the business [into early retirement] — people in their early fifties who have a nest egg."

Kelly also believes we might be headed toward a time when the social realities we face as a nation influence the type of physicians entering practice.

"I hate to talk about the economics, but it's something we struggle with. You talk about the perception of physicians. Today, if I see a physician driving a Honda Civic, I wonder. I drove a Toyota when I first started practice. That may get back to that gender thing. Women may be able to be happy making $95,000 a year as a pediatrician," he concluded, "but there's the perception that a good physician is a successful physician. And that means money."

DOES DREAM MEET REALITY?

Long-standing stereotypes don't die easily, including those that doctors make great money and are highly respected in the community; that they are their own bosses, conducting the day-to-day business of their profession with little supervision or second-guessing; and that once their long and rigorous training is over, they have it made and can prepare to spend their days involved in an intellectually challenging, lucrative, and satisfying career.

As has been illustrated so far in this book, and with recent studies backing it up, those ideas are showing their age. Beginning with America's health-care reform movement of the 1980s, the "givens" of a doctor's life have seen serious changes. By the 1990s, many doctors began to express deep levels of career dissatisfaction. As this century opened, a flurry of surveys began to appear, some showing that as many as 40 percent of doctors questioned said that, if they had it to do over again, they wouldn't choose medicine as a career.

The levels of and reasons for this dissatisfaction varied among individuals, areas of specialization, and geographic location, but across the board, respondents reported some common sources of frustration with the realities of medical practice in America. According to Bruce Landon, MD, of the Harvard Medical School, patient-care issues and relationships with patients and colleagues rank high in the factors physicians cite as contributing to workplace satisfaction, as do income and clinical autonomy — all of which have undergone a lot of change over the past few decades in ways that many of us just don't realize.

Let's start with what many in the public might consider to be one of the most attractive aspects of a career in medicine — a doctor's income. It's true that physicians are among the most well-paid professionals in the United States. In 2006, Physicians Search, a consultant to the health-care industry, listed average incomes for family practitioners at just over $145,500; for otolaryngologists, nearly $265,000; for cardiologists, $317,500; for radiologists, just over $347,000; and cardiovascular surgeon salaries averaged nearly $559,000. That's good money.

It's also true that, while doctors' salaries have risen over the past several years, they haven't kept up with "wage inflation" as have many other careers. According to a 2003 report published by the American Medical Association (AMA) titled "Physician Income: The Decade in Review," the median net annual income for all physicians in 2000 was $175,000 — an increase of just under 35 percent in the years following 1990. Over roughly the same period of time, the average American household income rose by 41 percent (from $35,225 to $49,600). The authors of the report, Carol K. Kane, PhD, and Horst Loeblich, also found that 75 percent of all physicians earned salaries under $250,000, and 25 percent earned less than $123,000 annually. In spite of gains in net income, real income for many doctors has been flat, or even diminished slightly over the past several years.

What plays a role in how much a doctor makes? Area of specialization is perhaps the most important factor. According to the Physicians Search figures cited above, average physician income can vary as much as $400,000 a year among specializations. However, seven of the twelve specialization areas highlighted in the AMA study experienced *decreases* in real income, and the largest hits were to salaries of surgical subspecialists and emergency medicine physicians.

Gender is another important factor in physician salary. In 2004, the U.S. Census Bureau reported that female physicians earned just sixty-three cents for every dollar earned by their male colleagues. Although women doctors diminished the gender gap in salary somewhat during the early 1990s, those gains were quickly lost; median income for this group dropped by 3.1 percent every year between 1995 and 2000. With more women joining the medical workforce, this means that more of our doctors are earning less every year.

Geographic location also plays an important role in how much a doctor earns. Kane's and Loeblich's research found the highest median income for doctors in the East and West South Central parts of the United States, and lowest in the Pacific and Mountain Regions. The price of real estate and other cost-of-living factors contribute to these differences, but the types of clients and service payers (private or public) and their reimbursement rates also play a role in how much money local doctors earn.

Finally, the cost of malpractice insurance (cited by many doctors as one of the biggest sources of career dissatisfaction) has gone up dramatically. A study published by the Massachusetts Medical Society found that, across the United States, the cost of professional liability insurance rose at an average annual rate of 63 percent each year from 1992 to 2003.

While physician salaries remain high, rising costs of doing business escalated at a much higher rate than did the median income for doctors. Between 1990 and 2000, when the costs of doing business for most physicians rose dramatically, physician median income increased, on average, by no more than 0.2 percent a year. Depending on their area of specialization, gender, geographic location, and other variables, physicians today *might* make great money, but they're more likely to be making *good* money performing a tough, demanding job.

As in most professions, money matters to many of the people who contemplate a career in medicine. One resident told us that many of her fellow students won't consider entering an area of specialization that can't guarantee an income of at least $200,000 a year. "They don't want to live on less than that," she stated.

WHERE DO DOCTORS GO FOR HELP?

Ironically, while doctors are more vulnerable to some of the stresses of modern life, they are actually *less* likely to seek and receive expert help in dealing with those issues. Denying our human vulnerabilities can damage us as individuals, but it's even more dangerous when it becomes common within a group that relies largely on peer review for regulation. If at times we sense that doctors think they're omnipotent, perhaps what we're actually experiencing is the doctors' fear that they must appear to be omnipotent in order to be taken seriously as physicians. When doctors feel that they must be considered infallible by others, their ability to honestly assess their own performance (or that of their colleagues) can be severely compromised.

As we've seen, to avoid any potential threat to their image of steadfast wellness, many doctors will attempt to self-diagnose and self-treat physical and emotional problems, rather than consult another doctor. When doctors *do* seek help from colleagues, they often don't receive unbiased treatment recommendations due to the stigma within the medical community surrounding doctor illness.

Physicians are inclined to extend "special treatment" to their peers, which frequently can translate into delayed or missed diagnoses or insufficient treatment for severe problems. Doctors can be reluctant, for example, to diagnose emotional problems in other physicians or recommend hospitalization for a severely depressed medical peer, knowing that such diagnoses might damage that person's career. As a result, physicians are at risk for receiving no treatment or the wrong kind of treatment for whatever illness they may be suffering. The adage "Doctor, heal thyself" holds some sad truth.

Seeking help, treatment, or even advice in the struggle with depression can feel like an admission of weakness; for women trying to establish their position within a competitive and still male-dominated profession, admitting to any kind of emotional problem can be especially difficult. In one example cited in the *Journal of Southern Medicine* study, a first-year resident in psychiatry suffered from depression, which robbed her of sleep and the ability to concentrate. She postponed getting psychiatric help because she didn't want to use her insurance and risk having others in her program find out she was having emotional problems (and remember, this woman was doing her residency *in psychiatry*). She also worried that a history of psychiatric treatment would inhibit her ability to get a medical license. (That worry wasn't unfounded, either; in many states, doctors with a recorded history of treatment for psychiatric disorders are subjected to increased scrutiny when considered for licensing.) The resident eventually entered counseling, but not before her problems had reached a critical stage. Within three weeks of beginning anti-depressant treatment, the young woman committed suicide.

TOMORROW'S PHYSICIAN SHORTAGE — TODAY

Our country is facing a shortage of trained physicians, but many Americans don't know it — with good reason. For the past twenty-five years, the American Medical Association insisted that America was actually suffering from a *surplus* of physicians. That reported surplus is used by both the government and the medical industry as a rationale for limiting the number of enrollees and graduates in medical schools across the nation. The AMA wasn't alone in its position: The Council on Graduate Medical Education (COGME) and the Association of American Medical Colleges (AAMC) also supported limitations on the number of new physicians, to stem the tide of what was portrayed as a potentially costly doctor surplus.

In 2005, however, all of this accepted wisdom turned upside-down with the release of a number of studies indicating a huge and growing shortage of physicians in America. If these studies are correct — and the AMA, Accreditation Council for Graduate Medical Education (ACGME), and AAMC all now agree that they are — we could find ourselves scrambling to fill 85,000 to 200,000 physician vacancies by the year 2020. To combat the shortage, we will need to train an additional 3,000 to 10,000 physicians annually. Obviously, because medical training takes a long time, we'd better start soon.

What happened to the "surplus"? In the 1960s and '70s, American medical colleges cranked out physicians in unprecedented numbers. Americans fund medical residencies, investing close to $110,000 in each newly licensed doctor. Congress, hungry to slash programs and save money in the 1980s, pointed to the high enrollment numbers of the preceding two decades as it voted to limit the number of paid medical residencies. Doctors weren't opposed to the limitations, either, as a controlled market offered more (and more lucrative) job opportunities for those students who made it into medical school.

Now, those doctors trained in the 1960s and '70s are retiring or cutting back on hours, just as fellow baby boomers reach an age of increased dependence on medical services. According to Richard Cooper, director of the Health Policy Institute at the Medical College of Wisconsin, "We face at least a decade of severe physician shortages because a bunch of people cooked numbers to support a position that was obviously wrong."

SICK OF DOCTORS?

Many experts have floated solutions for the pending shortage, including adding more residency slots in rural areas and small cities and increasing enrollment at medical schools. Between 2003 and 2007, first-year enrollment at America's 126 medical schools rose more than 7 percent, and 11 of those schools increased the sizes of their entering classes by more than 10 percent. These solutions require funding, of course, at both the state and federal level. Many communities are also seeking local solutions: Some hospitals and clinics in underserved areas offer student loan reimbursement and other incentives to doctors who will agree to practice in their area for a specified number of years.

Good news is on the horizon. Medical school enrollments in the United States hit an all-time high in 2007, with 17,800 first-year enrollees — a 2.3 percent increase over the previous year. The number of applicants that year grew by 8.2 percent over 2006. The same year saw an increase in the number of racial and ethnic minority applicants, as well, with the numbers of both black male and Hispanic male applicants increasing by 9.2 percent. The number of first-time applicants in 2007 was the highest on record with the AAMC.

We'll need these new doctors. By 2030, the number of Americans over the age of sixty-five is expected to be double what it was in 2000; at the same time, one of every three doctors currently in practice is expected to retire by the year 2020.

CHAPTER 11
PREPARE FOR THE FUTURE

RICHARD FELDMAN IS A PHYSICIAN who is well grounded in the realities of America's health-care struggles; he has practiced family medicine in Indiana for the past twenty-seven years, and he served as the Indiana State Health Commissioner from 1997–2001. Feldman's family history is rooted in the practice of medicine. His father was a family doctor who immigrated to the United States in 1920, then returned to Europe for medical training. He escaped the terrors of Nazi Germany and returned to this country, serving during World War II as a medical officer before embarking on a forty-five-year career in family medicine. Feldman gratefully acknowledges his father's influence on his own attitude and approach to medicine.

Although he remains deeply aware of the way medicine has evolved in America over the past century, Feldman also is actively involved in shaping the future of medicine through his work as director of the family medicine residency program at St. Francis Hospital in Beech Grove, Indiana, just south of Indianapolis. He also writes a monthly op/ed column for the *Indianapolis Star*, in which he discusses emerging health-care trends and issues in local, state, and national policy.

For the past several years, Feldman has been tracking — and writing about — many of the issues discussed in this book. One that he's followed most closely is consumer-driven health care. While Feldman sees rationale for this movement, he doesn't believe it's the solution to America's health-care ills.

ONE DOCTOR'S VISION FOR FUTURE HEALTH CARE

"One of the problems with our health-care system is that most people have first-dollar coverage," Feldman said. "When someone else is paying the bill, you don't care. You won't ask what an MRI costs or whether you really need it. Of course, doctors know that much of the testing they do is going to be negative; but medico-legally, it's necessary. This consumer-driven movement is designed to put patients in the consumer mode of looking at what these things cost and whether they need them.

"But a lot of people think this is the answer to our health-care system, and it's not. It's not going to cure the ills of our system. It's not going to extend health care to those who need it. In many ways, it doesn't even make sense. Are you going to shop around for the best price on an MRI? No, you're locked into a network. You have to go to certain hospitals to get it.

"The whole system of pricing is artificial anyway," Feldman continued. "Our health-care system doesn't follow the usual rule of economics. Prices are set based on what insurance pays; actually, they're set higher because everyone gets a discount. So shopping around isn't feasible.

"Do we want consumers asking themselves, 'Well . . . do I *really* need the test? Let me take my chances and see if I get worse, rather than spend a thousand dollars out of my pocket or health savings account.' So in terms of lowering health-care costs or making health-care dollars available to more people, it has a limited utility. The people who need insurance the most may not be sophisticated enough to manage a health savings account. Many of the working poor don't even have checking accounts. And I wonder — I don't want to sound like an elitist, but are these people capable of managing these accounts? And will they have the money to pay the high deductables?"

It's Feldman's opinion that Americans will need to avoid the "bargain-hunter" approach to health care that might be promoted by a move to health savings accounts (HSAs). "You have the combination of cost, quality, and value. What you want is best value — it may not be the cheapest and it may not be the very top quality, but somewhere in between you get the best value for your dollar. What consumer is going to be able to figure that out? I'm not convinced that HSAs will be the cure; they're a Band-Aid, a grand experiment, but for a number of reasons, not the answer.

"The answer is to be like the rest of the world; the rest of the world has government-subsidized health-care coverage for their populations. There's a price to pay for that, though. You have to give up something when you cover all people and make it affordable so everyone can get coverage. And you're going to see some policy changes regarding elderly people. If we get into a crisis of some sort, we'll create a system that won't pay for ninety-two-year-olds to get heart surgery or a hip replacement or renal dialysis or whatever. I'm not sure Americans are ready for rationing."

Feldman sees a need for broad reform in our national health-care system, rather than fixing individual aspects in piecemeal fashion. "Ours is a runaway system," Feldman asserted. "It's out of control — too much over-specialization. If you build these specialty hospitals, these heart hospitals and orthopedic hospitals, doctors and health networks will fill them up with paying patients. And let me tell you that few of these places specialize in treating ninety-year-olds with pneumonia. These competitors force community hospitals to have a fancy heart wing. As a result, we duplicate services and overspecialize, so we can generate more 'business.' Health care in America has become its own economic engine, and it's artificial and it's all going to collapse."

What is the first and most important step that could strengthen our national approach to health care? "First and foremost," Feldman responded, "we need universal health care. That doesn't necessarily mean single-payer insurance, but we need universal health care, and all people will have to pay into it. Right now, one-third of the uninsured in America *choose* not to be insured — for the most part, these are young, healthy people who don't think they need health care and don't want to pay for it. It's just like any other tax-base: if you have everybody paying in, you have more dollars to support those most in need of the service. Without that requirement you won't be able to afford or pay for the system."

Feldman elaborated on how the current system of private insurance plays a major role in the health-care quandary that exists today. "You have a lot of politics in this whole situation, which makes for a lot of personal inertia. And you have the insurance industry, which is very powerful, taking 20 percent to 40 percent of every health-care dollar. A lot of doctors are just sick of the whole thing. They're sick of the formularies, the paperwork, the rules, the oversight. The easiest payer segment to deal with right now is Medicare. You get paid — it's relatively straightforward. So a growing segment of doctors say, 'Let's just go with a government program and simplify our life.'"

He acknowledges the hazards that could evolve from both the consumer-driven health-care movement and the idea of a single-payer, Medicare-like system. "Once Medicare has the whole population as a captive audience, things could change dramatically. Consider, for example, the current pay-for-performance movement. There's nothing inherently wrong with pay-for-performance, but it's nearly impossible to do it right. In some ways, it's an irrational system that's grown from Medicare; nevertheless, it is gaining interest within some hospitals, employers, and health plans. Many private groups, too, are deciding that they would prefer to pay more for quality care.

"But, back to the future," Feldman continued. "I think health care will become a combination of private insurance and government assistance. Since single-payer won't fly (unless we have a real crisis); I think you'll see what some states are doing, but on a national level. We'll pool our Medicaid money, our Medicare money, and all the tax subsidies we give employers now for providing health insurance, subsidize that amount with a broad-based tax, and use the combined funds to create a basic health-care policy for all Americans. Everyone will be able to use that coverage to go in and get basic preventive care and catastrophic care. In the middle will be the private sector, which will make the whole thing fly. The middle class and upper class will have the opportunity to buy additional coverage for more personalized, efficient, or timely care. They'll pay for it through

WOULD "PAY FOR PERFORMANCE" GUARANTEE GOOD OUTCOMES?

As Richard Feldman, MD, sees it, the problem with pay-for-performance — a system that rewards doctors and medical services institutions based on patient outcomes — is finding adequate measures. "There are two types of measures — process and outcome. I don't have a problem with process concentration: Did you tell patients things they need to know? Did you follow the recommended interventions? Did you run the recommended tests, periodic checks, and so on? All these things are evidence-based aspects of good medical service. So it's proper process to order a test twice a year, or to tell a patient to see an ophthalmologist once a year, or to recommend strategies to get blood pressure down.

"*Outcomes*, however, depend on patient compliance and you have a lot of patients who are noncompliant. If you judge me on a patient's hemoglobin count [a red-blood-cell profile], well . . . I'm doing my best, but that doesn't mean the patient will comply with my recommendations. If I'm in private practice and I'm going to get paid more based on outcomes, then I'll dump the noncompliant and the sickest patients. And that's not a workable system. Judging doctors on outcomes is a slippery slope. How do you even find out whether I'm giving good recommendations? Right now, it's all tied to billing, so if a lab has a billing for a blood test, then the doctor did his part."

premiums, I think, that will be a combination of employer or private coverage for everyone.

"Of course, the insurance industry won't like this plan, either, and they're a very powerful entity. For all I know, they'll run the government program — they could. Of course, Medicare runs itself, and that would be the way to go because you'd have very low overhead. But as long as the individuals who can afford it can buy additional coverage and more services, and get to the front of the line, I think it will be politically feasible. The result will be a tiered system, which we already have. Some people can afford a Chevrolet, and some can afford a Rolls Royce, and that's just the way the system is. But as long as everyone can get basic care, that's an important step."

Could the economic incentive of reducing public health-care costs spur more compliance with the practices of healthy living? Feldman isn't convinced that a commitment to universal health care could trigger a widespread interest in health maintenance in this country. "Half of my career is in public health," he noted, "and this country is more than willing to pay billions of dollars to treat diseases, but it's incredible how little we are willing to pay to prevent them. I've constantly fought for adequate prevention/cessation programs for tobacco. When I began as State Health Commissioner, Indiana's smoking rate was at 27 percent; today, nearly ten years later, it remains at about 27 percent.

"We need a cultural change in America. I think 2 percent of our dollars are spent on public health, and I don't see any movement in this country toward greater consciousness of public health. Public health is a public good, rather than an individual good: it affects all people, but we don't realize it when we benefit from it. We don't worry about the food we eat or the water we drink; safeguarding all these things is done for everyone, and it's completely invisible. It's only when we get a crisis like West Nile, SARS, or other epidemics, that we care about disease prevention. One hundred years ago, acute infectious diseases were what killed people — smallpox, scarlet fever, typhoid, and so on. We conquered those and we now live longer and die of chronic diseases, which take decades to unfold. No one sees immediate benefit from combating those types of public health issues, so they don't care."

Nevertheless, Feldman agrees that economic incentives are tied into the whole idea of universal health care. "Yes, the public health movement has tried to use that recently. They don't go for the idea of, hey, it's going to improve your health. They emphasize the cost of poor prevention practices. So what we've done now is concentrate on costs; we spend $2 billion a year on tobacco-related health problems in Indiana, and employers here spend another $1.4 billion on tobacco-related issues: lost time, reduced productivity, and so on. We have those economics worked out because politically we feel that's a stronger motivator [for funding programs such as smoking cessation and public education] than improving the health of people.

"There's a huge synergy when you combine health-care policy and public-health policy — and there are efforts to combine those things. More and more employers are trying to have wellness programs and are funding stop-smoking programs. There is a growing awareness of the costs of chronic disease."

Feldman sees some possibility that a move toward universally funded health care might help close the gap between doctors and patients by reviving the notion that doctors are more concerned with their patients' best interests than with issues of their own wealth, power, and prestige.

"I hate to admit it," he said, "and the medical profession doesn't like to talk about it, but I think there's been a decrease in professionalism in medicine — especially among certain specialties — even since I've come into practice. Today, as a family physician, it can be hard to find a specialist who will take care of a Medicaid patient. The specialists — the neurosurgeon, the orthopedic surgeon — want to be paid to be on call for the hospital, for the emergency department, wherever they can make the most. When I first went into practice, if I had a patient without money, the specialists I referred to would say, 'I'll take all your patients.' That was the standard. It's not that way anymore.

"But," he was quick to add, "make no mistake, there's still a lot of altruism in medicine. You have a lot of family doctors, especially in rural communities, who lose money every time they see a Medicaid patient, but they feel that they are part of the community, and it's part of their duty to provide that community service. It gets harder every year, but don't ever discount the altruism remaining in medicine.

"We've gotten where we are because doctors are working harder to make less money or to just stay even. Priorities change. Almost nobody's going into family medicine in Indiana, for example. We've seen a 50 percent decrease in applicants because everyone is specializing. If we just say we need more doctors, we're ignoring the complete picture. We need policy that specifically will create more primary-care physicians. We have shortages of cardiologists and other specialties too, but that's because of this artificial system. You can't look at what we'll need in the future based on what we have now; still, it's obvious that we need more primary care. That's the basis of quality medicine — and it's being left behind."

FAMILY DOCTORS

In spite of his awareness of the challenges facing America in reshaping its national health-care policies, when he shifts his focus to the day-to-day workings of the individual doctor–patient relationships that make up that massive system, Feldman remains hopeful about the future. "Day in and day out," he said, "I have wonderful relationships with our patients. I think they trust me and I enjoy seeing them. And that type of doctor–patient relationship still happens, especially in the smaller towns. Those doctors are treating their friends and neighbors. Given the chance, I think that things could be like they were years ago, and that medicine will triumph again.

"The corporatization of medicine has damaged that; and the new docs coming out don't know anything different. We teach all the right principles, but in practice, these new residents don't know anything different than the system they've grown up with. Given the chance, though, I think that family docs will reconnect with their patients and know them as individuals and develop those long-term relationships that result in quality care."

In writing about the importance of family doctors in America today, Richard Feldman has paid tribute to his father and the other mid-twentieth-century general practitioners who helped form this country's proudest era of medical care. "He called himself a general practitioner," Feldman wrote of his father in an editorial for the *Indianapolis Star*. "The principles of comprehensive and continuous personalized patient care came to him and other general practitioners of his generation by experience and sensitivity to the needs of their patients."

In conclusion, Feldman noted that family doctors "continue to be the heart and soul of medicine. More than any other specialty, family doctors humanize the health-care experience. Focusing their attention on the person, not just the disease, they are driven by the need to make people whole."

DOCTORS FALL OFF THEIR PEDESTALS

More Americans now are realizing the value of those relationships Feldman described above, even if fewer of them have the means or ability to achieve them. Still, we are making strides toward repairing the past few decades of damage to the practice of medicine and those relationships. This is an exciting time in our nation's health-care history, with possibilities for growth and change that stretch well beyond our imaginations. Some of the best news, however, is that each one of us, individually, will play a key role in shaping our medical future.

The old order has changed. Our doctors have been toppled from their pedestals by a natural evolution of the way we need and use health care in this country, and we patients are on a different footing, too. Medicine was our greatest weapon against infectious disease, and — to a great extent — those battles are won. In the fight against chronic diseases and problems of aging, however, we need a different arsenal of tools, such as preventive care, a healthy lifestyle, and proactive maintenance. Most important, we need a strong working relationship with the men and women of medicine.

It's easy to feel lost in all of the ongoing debates and conflicting ideas about how to solve our national health-care crisis. In the end, however, none of these big ideas and institutions really matter as much to each of us individually as what happens when our doctor steps into the examining room. Will our doctor give us a thorough examination, listen to our concerns, keep an open mind, answer our questions, and discuss our options with us? In other words, will we be a whole, human being or simply a "condition" to be dealt with and dismissed as quickly as possible? The answers to those questions will determine how well we've solved our own individual issues of health-care reform.

No, we cannot turn back the clock. America will never be the country it was a century ago, and few of us would want to forego the medical and social advancements made in that time. Most of us will live longer, healthier lives than any generation in history, and we'll be counting on our doctors to help make our extended years pleasant and productive. We can be glad that Doctor God is dead and that the cycle of medicine in America is entering a new phase that is likely to be the best one yet. Sure, we have some work to do, but we have a lot to look forward to as well.

THE EVOLUTION OF HEALTH CARE

When this project began, I spent a lot of time explaining the topic of the book to friends, family, and potential interviewees. Most people seemed truly excited about the notion of exploring the topic of health care, and many of those folks assumed *someone* would be raked over the coals. Whether the presumed culprits are doctors, hospitals, managed-care programs, the government, Medicaid, Medicare, the insurance industry, malpractice lawyers, or people who bleed the system with medical malingering or frivolous lawsuits — you name it — most people have identified at least one group, class, company, or organization that is to blame for the disheveled state of our nation's health-care system. In an age where any call to accountability is dismissed (at least, by the guilty party) as "playing the blame game," many Americans are downright thirsty to take someone to task for one of our country's most costly and damaging ills. If we can determine who's responsible for this mess, maybe we can make them clean it up — right?

In the final analysis, though, there is no villain in the story of America's health-care crisis. What was discovered — and what I hope is made clear by the information included in this book — is that *all* of us bear some responsibility for the state of medicine today.

Take doctors, for example. For too long, the MDs operated in a rarified atmosphere of arrogance, power, and control that isolated them from their patients and their own humanity. In their all-consuming desire to avoid governmental control, doctors willingly stepped into the yoke of corporate oversight, trading their future autonomy — and their patients' ultimate welfare — for the fat and easy salad days of the medical insurance industry boom.

And what about the insurance industry? Today, the benefits of our medical system are for all practical purposes managed and dispensed by that industry, which enjoys record profits even as it sometimes refuses to grant benefits to people for the conditions that render them most needy of insurance in the first place. Health-care insurance premiums have risen more than 75 percent since the year 2000 and more than 50 percent faster than inflation. Insurance companies aren't the only corporate players in this game; many of America's largest corporations — including some in the health-care industry — contributed to our nation's health-care woes by severely limiting their support for employee health-care programs in order to bolster profits. And as medical errors continue to rise, too many hospital CEOs worry more about their financial viability than they do about the quality of care in their institutions.

Then there's us, the American people. By abdicating all responsibility for managing our health care and tracking its expenses, we patients helped dig ourselves into this medical mess. We like to complain about our doctors acting like gods, but we were only too happy to sit back and let them assume that role. With an insurance company picking up the tab, why should we bother asking why we needed that test or prescription, three follow-up appointments, or the services of a specialist — or how much any of that would cost? Well, those days are over. Today, in a time when medical technology is at its zenith (and driving up the cost of health care in this country), millions of Americans are left scrambling to find ways to pay for even the most basic care. For them it matters a great deal what those X-rays will cost or whether they really need to take those antibiotics as they recover from a cold.

Our lifestyles have caught up with us, too. For too long, we Americans made little effort to maintain our long-term health. We let fast-food restaurants take over our school cafeterias, even as those same schools dropped physical education programs. We eagerly rewarded innovations such as larger automobile cup-holders and more drive-thru windows, and ignored the decline of neighborhood sidewalks and public parks. Even today, with mounting evidence that we can't afford to prop up unhealthy lifestyles with heroic medical intervention, we're more interested in fixing our health care system than we are in fixing our unhealthy way of living.

But if most of us can simply look in the mirror to find someone responsible for the state of medicine today, we'll see someone who has the power to help straighten out the mess. More Americans than ever before are united in their determination to find a workable solution to our nation's health care woes. In this book, you've read about many of their efforts. Our colleges and universities are changing the way they teach medicine, to make doctors more responsive to and engaged with their patients, and to create a more humane approach to the practice of medicine. Hospitals are adopting programs and procedures to help improve patient safety, promote a team approach to medicine, and avoid breakdowns in communication.

Federal, state, and local governments are answering citizen demands for change too. Public policies are bolstering efforts to promote healthier living; even cities in tobacco-belt states like

Kentucky have adopted smoking bans to help rid public spaces of second-hand smoke. Many of our school systems have given soft-drink and fast-food vendors the boot, and are promoting healthier food choices and increased exercise through concrete programs, rather than merely paying lip service to benefits of physical fitness. Some insurance companies have begun offering increased coverage for preventive care and healthy lifestyle programs. And, as you who bought this book know, Americans are paying more attention to issues of both personal and public health as they shoulder more of the responsibility for dealing with the impact of those issues.

All of these changes are altering the landscape of medicine in this country in ways that we might not yet fully understand or appreciate. We and our doctors face the task of developing new approaches to deal with the evolving realities of health care in America. It's just as important that we recognize that our system never stops evolving. Now, more than ever, we patients need to understand the way our system works (and doesn't work), and the possibilities of the many developments taking shape on America's health-care horizon.

Being of sound mind and body at age seventy-five justifies, I think, my ruminating about an earlier era of doctor-hero worship. The trust exhibited by patients toward their physicians years ago was akin to a really good marital relationship. But when it's over, it's over.

Today, I have different expectations. For example, whenever I have a "first date" with a new doctor I am well prepared, even having a print-out that lists allergies, personal and family medical history, all medical incidents, drugs and supplements I take. It's more than helpful for the doctor, and I can be sure I don't forget something that could have an impact on my treatment.

The way medicine was practiced when I was born in 1934 is certainly different from how it is today. I'm pleased for the most part with how the field has evolved and my own understanding of the choices available to me. Nevertheless, I often wonder where medicine will be in five, ten, twenty years, and considering the advances today's rapidly changing technology offers, I realize that the future is *now*.

SICK OF DOCTORS?

As stated in the first chapter, at the beginning of the twentieth century, doctors across the United States enjoyed a prominent status within their communities and earned a respectable income. Most had long-term relationships with the families they treated; they traveled to patients' homes for most services and often charged fees in keeping with the family's ability to pay, at times even accepting bartered goods in exchange for their services.

Those were the days before the AMA emerged and the government set rules and regulations for medical practitioners. By the time World War II ended, medicine had become more "industrialized," moving away from home-based care and offering physicians more prestige, power, and wealth than ever before. Salaries skyrocketed, third-party payer insurance buffered most patients and doctors from the charges for medical services, and powerful corporate interests stepped in to help drive profits even higher. The number and types of doctors we saw grew larger while our appointment times grew shorter.

A great number of Americans began to resent the almost factory-like approach to health care that over time became the norm. The good old family doc went the way of the dinosaur, and we were left to deal with the dreaded Doctor God.

The cycle was still in motion. Insurance oversight eclipsed doctors' authority and medical institutions scrambled to compete for shrinking payment dollars. Health maintenance organizations, with their managed-care approach, limited health-care access for many Americans and completely transformed the medical workplace and the doctor–patient relationship. Insurance costs skyrocketed and more and more Americans found themselves without coverage; some couldn't afford the premiums and others chose not to pay them. Everyone — doctors and patients alike — struggled to find ways to deal with a system that seemed to offer no one the benefits of a sound, affordable, and effective approach to health care.

Where we stand today is in many ways an unattractive spot. Most modern medical facilities are run like any other corporation, with the primary focus on the bottom line. Services that fail to produce sufficient revenue are cut and resources are devoted to areas where profits are more reasonably assured. Some doctors feel betrayed: salaries for most aren't as generous as they used to be, paperwork and administrative duties consume ever more time, and insurance companies — not doctors — call the shots when it comes to determining who is eligible to receive specific treatments.

Furthermore, many experienced doctors are retiring early to avoid the realities of life as an employee of a bureaucratic system. Frustration with poor working conditions, low pay, and flagging morale is taking a toll on other medical staff, too. Nurses also are retiring early and fewer people are entering the field. Couple these trends with America's aging population and we may be looking at a perfect storm of medical difficulties.

We need to rethink our whole approach to health care in this country, but to a great extent, that kind of change begins one citizen at a time. Fundamentally, we — each of us — will begin the process of reinventing it by changing the way we work with our doctors. Ideally, we will come up with a system that incorporates the best of what has been good about American health care in the past with the rapidly changing benefits of emerging trends and technologies. To do it right, though, we'll need to avoid the attitudes and practices and prejudices that have made our system so dysfunctional and realize that sound solutions rest on a foundation of personal responsibility — for staying healthy, red-flagging developing medical conditions, and seeking prompt treatment for those diseases and illnesses that we cannot ward off.

Taking charge is good for both the health of our bodies and our pocketbooks. When we manage our diabetes at home, use home-testing to eliminate or confirm initial diagnoses, or take care of a sick or elderly family member in our own homes, we dramatically reduce our medical expenses. At the same time, we're easing the strain on our medical system and freeing up doctors, facilities, and equipment to deal with others whose conditions aren't right for home-based care. Reducing medical expenses also (in theory, at least) can reduce the costs of medical insurance, as lower expenditures translate into slower premium hikes. A movement toward more home-based care also could result in better public education about health issues that could result in helping us all to live healthier lives and to become better prepared to step up when we or a family member needs basic care.

As America looks closer at the ideas of universal health-care coverage, one notion we will have to embrace is the idea that we can't afford to ignore the impact of unhealthy lifestyles. We're a nation of fierce individualism, but when our medical "fortunes" are tied together, we'll be united in finding ways to combat the causes and contributors to major health problems in our country. It's unknown yet what all of these developments will mean for health care in America, but it's a pretty safe bet that good things lie ahead.

Resources

Following are some helpful resources available to those seeking more information about the topics discussed in this book, particularly regarding patient empowerment. Many of the books listed in the Bibliography offer their own lists of resources, as well.

Consumer Information and Patient Safety Tips

The Agency for Healthcare Research and Quality (AHRQ) website (sponsored by the United States Department of Health and Human Services) offers a variety of information and resources for medical consumers, including consumer versions of clinical practice guidelines, questions to ask your medical team prior to surgery, and next-step guides for those who have been diagnosed with common health conditions and diseases. Visit the site at www.ahrq.gov.

The AHRQ also offers a wealth of information on the topics of medical errors and patient safety. To access the agency's tip sheets for preventing medical errors, safe practices for better health care, and patient safety tools and resources, visit the agency's main web page (www.ahrq.gov), then choose Medical Errors & Patient Safety from the Quality and Patient Safety listing.

The Patient Advocacy Foundation (PAF) is a nationwide, nonprofit organization formed to help individuals experiencing problems associated with health care, including advice for gaining access to care, maintaining employment and financial stability during a health-care crisis or long-term treatment program. Their website (www. patientadvocate.org) offers links to a number of helpful resources, as well as announcement of upcoming programs and emerging issues in medical care.

SICK OF DOCTORS?

The Robert Wood Johnson Foundation is a private, philanthropic organization dedicated to helping improve health and health care in America. The organization's website carries valuable information about innovative programs, legislation, new research, and educational opportunities related to health care in America. To learn more, visit the website at http://rwjf.org, or contact the organization at:

RWJF 2007

P.O. Box 2316 College Road East and Route 1

Princeton, NJ 08543

(888) 631-9989

COMPARE HOSPITALS

Another site associated with the AHRQ, the Hospital Compare online tool, allows you to search for hospitals by name, zip code, or other geographic locator, and then compare those hospitals' performance on major medical issues such as heart attack, pneumonia, and infections. This sophisticated program provides plenty of customizable search options — a great tool for checking and comparing the quality of hospitals in your area. Visit www.hospitalcompare.hhs.gov/

The Joint Commission (www.jointcommission.org) is an accreditation and standards organization that accredits over 15,000 U.S. health-care organizations and programs. The Joint Commission's website offers links to a number of patient safety resources, as well as a searchable guide to Joint Commission-accredited hospitals and health-care facilities (available at http://www.jointcommission.org/GeneralPublic).

FIND A QUALIFIED DOCTOR

The American Medical Association website offers a "DoctorFinder" feature that you can use to search for information about physicians based on physician name and/or specialty and location. Access the feature at http://webapps.ama-assn.org/doctorfinder/html/patient.html

Resources

The American Board of Medical Specialties (ABMS) oversees the standards of 24 different medical specialty boards. The ABMS website can be accessed at http://www.abms.org. Click the "Consumers" link on the ABMS home page to access links that will help you check the certification status of your own doctor (the service is free, but requires a login and password). The site also offers links to the individual certifying boards for each of the 24 medical specialties monitored by the ABMS. If you don't have online access, you can submit a written request for information to the ABMS at:

American Board of Medical Specialties
1007 Church Street, Suite 404
Evanston, IL 60201-5913

If you'd like to check your doctor's certification status by telephone, you can call toll-free 1-866-ASK-ABMS (275-2267.) This service provides certification status information only. If you'd like professional and biographical details about your doctor, you can check *The Official ABMS Directory of Board Certified Medical Specialists*, which is available in most public libraries.

The American College of Surgeons website offers a guide for choosing a qualified surgeon and answers to many common questions from those preparing to undergo a surgical procedure. Go to the main web page at www.facs.org, then choose the Public and Press Link to access the Find a Qualified Surgeon option.

CHECK THE LICENSING STATUS OF YOUR DOCTOR

All reputable doctors are licensed by their state medical licensing boards (osteopaths are licensed by state boards of osteopathic medicine). Through these boards, you can determine whether your doctor is licensed, and find out whether he or she has been disciplined by the state board. Links to medical licensing boards in all fifty states are available at the American Medical Association's

(AMA) public information page: http://www.ama-assn.org/ama/pub/category/2645.html

LEARN MORE ABOUT HEALTH INSURANCE AND HEALTH-CARE REFORM

The National Coalition on Health Care's guide to health insurance costs is offered online at www.nchc.org/facts/cost.shtml

Sponsored by the AMA, the Patients'ActionNetwork offers news, issues coverage, and a resource kit for advocates of health care reform (www.patientsactionnetwork.com).

The Health Insurance Association of America offers an online guide to health insurance, in all its many forms, posted by the Federal Citizen Information Center at www.pueblo.gsa.gov/cic_text/health/guidehealth/guidehealth.htm

The Robert Wood Johnson Foundation's website is devoted to the topic of health insurance coverage for all Americans. The Foundation is committed to working to make sure all Americans have reliable and affordable health insurance coverage by 2010. See what the organization has learned and follow its continuing efforts (including its annual Cover the Uninsured Week activities) at http://rwjf.org/portfolios/interestarea.jsp?iaid=132
    Online Healthcare Resources
    Research Health Conditions and Diseases
    Medline Plus, a website sponsored by the National Library of Medicine and the National Institutes of Health (NIH) offers an authoritative guide to over 700 health topics, drugs and supplements, and current health news. The site also provides a medical encyclopedia and dictionary, and links to finding health resources in your area. Visit the site at http://medlineplus.gov

The United States Department of Health and Human Services

Resources

(HHS) also sponsors a health-topic search engine that provides access to information on a wide range of diseases, conditions, and injuries, a drug database, and a guide to health-care organizations and agencies. Visit the site at www.healthfinder.gov.

CREATE AND MAINTAIN YOUR PERSONAL HEALTH RECORD

You can provide any physician or health-care agency a complete and accurate record of your medical history anywhere and at any time when you maintain your own personal health record. Learn more about the benefits of doing so, and find a step-by-step guide for creating and maintaining your record (on paper, in electronic form, or online) at the My Personal Health Record website (www.myphr. com/), hosted by the American Health Information Management Association (AHIMA).

The HHS Family History Initiative website also offers helpful information and guides for compiling your family health history, as well as a link to downloadable software designed to make the process simple and enjoyable. Visit that site at www.hhs.gov/familyhistory.

LEARN MORE ABOUT COMPLEMENTARY AND ALTERNATIVE MEDICINE

The National Center for Complementary and Alternative Medicine website, www.nccam.nih.gov, offers definitions, descriptions, and helpful guides to alternative and complementary medicine. You also can write to them at:

The National Center for Complementary
and Alternative Medicine
National Institutes of Health
9000 Rockville Pike
Bethesda, MD, 20892

BIBLIOGRAPHY

Banja, John, PhD. *Medical Errors and Medical Narcissism*. Sudbury, MA: Jones and Bartlett Publishers, 2004.

Committee on the Use of Complementary and Alternative Medicine by the American Public. *Complementary and Alternative Medicine in the United States*. Washington, DC: National Academy of Sciences, 2005.

Crenner, Christopher. *Private Practice: In the Early Twentieth-Century Medical Office of Dr. Richard Cabot*. Baltimore: Johns Hopkins University Press, 2005.

Evans, G., and N.L. Farberow, Kennedy Associates, eds. *The Encyclopedia of Suicide*, 2nd ed. New York: Facts on File, 2003.

Gawande, Atul, MD. *Complications*. New York: Picador Press, 2002.

Ginzberg, Eli, and Miriam Ostow. *The Coming Physician Surplus*. Totowa, NJ: Rowman and Allenheld, 1984.

Goleman, Daniel. *Social Intelligence: The New Science of Human Relationships*. New York: Bantam Books, 2006.

Gordon, Suzanne, *Nursing Against the Odds: How Health Care Cost Cutting, Media Stereotypes, and Medical Hubris Undermine Nurses and Patient Care*. Ithaca, NY, and London: ILR Press, 2005.

Hancock, David. *The Complete Medical Tourist*. London: John Blake Publishing, LTD, March 2006.

IOM Health Care Quality Initiative. *The Chasm in Quality: Select Indicators from Recent Reports*. Washington, DC: Institute of Medicine, 2006.

Kohn, Linda T., Janet M. Corrigan, and Molla S. Donaldson, eds. *To Err is Human: Building a Safer Health System*. Washington, DC: Committee on Quality of Health Care in America, Institute of Medicine, November 1999.

Konner, Melvin. *Medicine at the Crossroads*. New York: Pantheon Books, 1993.

Korsch, Barbara M., and C. Harding. *The Intelligent Patient's Guide to the Doctor-Patient Relationship*. New York: Oxford University Press, 1998.

Kovner, Anthony, and Steven Jonas. *Jonas and Kovner's Health Care Delivery in the United States*, 7th ed. New York: Springer Publishing Company, 2002.

Bibliography

Lown, Bernard, MD. *The Lost Art of Healing*. New York: Houghton Mifflin Company, 1996.

Ludmerer, Kenneth M., *Learning to Heal: The Development of American Medical Education*. Baltimore: Johns Hopkins University Press, 1996.

———. *Time to Heal: American Medical Education from the Turn of the Century to the Era of Managed Care*. New York: Oxford University Press, 1999.

Marion, Robert, MD. *Learning to Play God*. New York: Addison-Wesley Publishing Company, 1991.

———. *The Intern Blues*. New York: William Morrow and Company, 1989

McGregor-Robinson, J. *The Household Physician*. London: Gresham Publishing, 1902.

More, E.S., and M.A. Milligan, eds. *The Empathic Practitioner: Empathy, Gender and Medicine*. Piscataway, NJ: Rutgers University Press, 1994.

Myers, Michael F. *Doctors' Marriages: A Look at their Problems and Solutions*, 2nd ed. New York and London: Plenum Medical Book Co., 1994.

Nitzberg, Esther. *Hippocrates' Handmaidens: Women Married to Physicians*. New York and London: The Haworth Press, 1994.

O'Conner, P.G., and A. Spickard. *Physician Impairment by Substance Abuse*. Nashville, TN: Vanderbilt University Medical Center, 2001.

Preston, Thomas A., MD. *The Clay Pedestal: A Renowned Cardiologist Reexamines the Doctor-Patient Relationship*. New York: Charles Scribner's Sons, 1986.

Reina, Dennis and Michelle. *Trust and Betrayal in the Workplace*. San Francisco: Berrett-Koehler Publishers, 1999.

Robinson, James C. *The Corporate Practice of Medicine*. Los Angeles: University of California Press, 1999.

Rodwin, Marc A. *Medicine, Money, and Morals: Physicians' Conflicts of Interest*. New York: Oxford University Press, 1993.

Roizen, Michael, MD, and Mehmet C.Oz, MD, with the Joint Commission. *You: The Smart Patient: An Insider's Handbook for Getting the Best Treatment*. New York: Free Press, 2006.

Roter, Debra, PhD, and Judith Hall, PhD. *Doctors Talking with Patients/ Patients Talking with Doctors: Improving Communication in Medical Visits*. Westport, CT: Auburn House, 1992.

Shem, Samuel. *The House of God*. New York: Random House, 1975.

Sotile, Wayne M., PhD, and Mary O. Sotile, MA. *The Medical Marriage: Sustaining Healthy Relationships for Physicians and Their Families*, rev. ed. American Medical Association, 2000.

Starr, Paul. *The Social Transformation of Medicine in America*. New York: Basic Books, Inc., Harper Colophon Books, 1982.

Stewart, James B. *Blind Eye: How the Medical Establishment Let a Doctor Get Away with Murder*. New York: Simon and Schuster, 1999.

Sultz, Harry and Kristina M.Young. *Health Care USA: Understanding its Organization and Delivery*, 4th ed. Sudbury, MA: Jones and Bartlett Publishers, 2004.

Todd, Alexander; *Intimate Adversaries: Cultural Conflicts Between Doctors and Women Patients*. Philadelphia: University of Pennsylvania Press, 1989.

Toombs, Kay, PhD. *The Meaning of Illness: A Phenomenological Account of the Different Perspectives of Physician and Patient*. Norwell, MA: Kluwer Academic Publishers, 1992.

Wachter, Robert M., MD, and Kaveh Shojania, MD. *Internal Bleeding: The Truth Behind America's Terrifying Epidemic of Medical Mistakes*. New York: Rugged Land, 2004.